Wellness Toolbox

Debunking Myths About Fitness and Nutrition to Provide All the Tools You Need for a Healthier and Happier Life

Don Roberts

Fitness and Nutrition Specialist

First Edition

Cover design by Vanessa Mendozzi

Cartoons by Glasbergen

ISBN 9781790431984

Praise for Wellness Toolbox...

"Wonderful book – changed my life!" – M. Holland

"Helped me lose 60 pounds in 6 months." – D. Mortensen

"Science and real world application." – T. Quinn

"One of the most accurate and precise books..." – R. Robinson

"Something for everyone in this book." – S. Off

"Concise, well researched and very practical." – B. Wiggs

"So inspirational!" – D. Rodman

"Packed full of valuable information." – C. Long

"Excellent as a thorough resource." – A. Suran

"I will refer to it time and time again..." – J. Dickens

"Should be required reading in school." – J. Hamilton

"Easy, yet super informative. I love this book!" – M. Bush

"Great read! Great data! Super helpful!" – C. Macluskie

"Big fan of this book!" – C. Choate

"Highly recommended!" – P. Fitzgerald

"Great source of fitness and nutrition advice." – M. Garcia

"A must read for a healthy life." – C. Gill

Dedication

This book is dedicated to all of the individuals who have struggled over the years with diets and exercise programs, despite their diligent efforts. Most people have either been uninformed or misinformed in their quest for health. May this help you on your road to success.

Contents

Foreword

We live in very interesting times. All the information we want or sometimes don't even want, is literally at our fingertips at a moment's notice. We are bombarded with information of all types, particularly guidance on health and wellness and emphasizing the "should and should nots." How do we sort through all of this advice? How do we make good decisions about our health based on what we read? It can be extremely confusing given how much new information comes out regularly, how much of that is often conflicting, and the fact that health tips can be written or posted by persons with no real backing or research to support it.

I have personally worked in the wellness industry for over 25 years with a spectrum of responsibilities and roles. As a Holistic Wellness Coach, I sometimes struggle with distilling information properly to my clients, as they often read and hear a lot of conflicting reports and quickly become overwhelmed. It is very easy to become frustrated and confused, but one thing I come back to regularly is not getting caught up in the hype and fads, and to ask the following questions: Who is stating the information? Is there research to back it up? Who is funding the research? And most importantly, do not believe everything you hear. Do your homework, and definitely become your own advocate.

I have known Don Roberts for nearly 20 years, working with him at his Fitness Solutions 24/7 gym for much of that time. Throughout the years, Don has been a pillar of knowledge in the health and wellness industry, helping to educate and dispel myths to hundreds of people in and around our Durango community. I believe it is the perfect time for a book like this - an authoritative resource that can help us decipher between truths and myths in the world of fitness and nutrition. Don is sharing decades of experience and education. He explains fact versus fiction with thoughtful explanations, while breaking down the research to support it, thus making it much easier for people to sift through and incorporate the best and most relevant health information and practices into their lives. What a great tool to add to your health and wellness toolbox!

Enjoy and live well!

Lisa Nielsen
Holistic Health and Wellness Coach
www.viblifewellness.com

Preface

As a toddler, I was an active little fella. Growing up on a small ranch five miles east of Del Norte, Colorado, our long dirt road, alfalfa fields, grass pastures, old wooden barn and sheds, ditches, creek, river, cottonwood trees, and haystack made for a marvelous assortment of outdoor activities like running, climbing, jumping, swimming, ice skating, and playing. As the youngest of seven children, I most certainly kept my parents and siblings on their toes. Little did I know at the time that our property had provided me one of the finest recreational areas a kid could ever ask for.

Later, in grade school, whether playing baseball, football, basketball, racing around the playground, or riding my bicycle several miles at a time, I thoroughly enjoyed being active. I learned early on that exercise made me feel better mentally and physically.

Physical work around the ranch was part of my daily chores. Whether hauling, splitting, and stacking wood; building or repairing fences; irrigating; tending to livestock, and more, I was beginning to strengthen my scrawny muscles and weak bones, as well as develop my work ethic into my adolescence.

Unfortunately, as a young teenager, I made some rather poor choices. One of these choices got me into some trouble with the law and nearly cost me and others our lives. It was a difficult time to say the least.

A friend, my nephew, and I took my father's truck for a joy ride in the middle of the night to the neighboring town of Alamosa, about thirty miles away. With nothing happening in that town at 3:00 am, we decided to head home. Not knowing I had crossed a double yellow line exiting town, a police officer had us in his sight. With the bright red and blue lights flashing in the rear view mirror, I panicked. "I have to get us out of this situation or my parents are going to kill me!" was my only focus.

A high speed chase ensued for nearly twenty miles. Lots of cat and mouse antics followed for what seemed like hours, but was merely minutes. A roadblock was strategically positioned ahead, but was not effective as we swerved around it and onward. Multiple patrol cars from several departments (city, county, and state) now lit up the sky behind us. At this point, I had to be dreaming, right?

Unabated, the chaos continued down an unfamiliar and narrow dirt road. We made a hard left turn. The speed was just too much. We hit a dirt embankment on the side of the road and became airborne. Rolling and flipping some 150-odd-feet, the truck finally came to a stop. Shocked, but uninjured, the three of us were pulled out of the mangled truck.

Handcuffed and placed in the back of a Colorado State Troopers car, we headed to the Alamosa County Jail. Albeit only fourteen years old, I was given multiple citations.

Those actions nearly landed me in a detention center, not to mention the morgue. Community service for two years was part of my punishment, along with extra hard work around our ranch. Throughout it all, faith, family, friends, fitness, and food (pardon all the "f's") allowed me to stay grounded and happy. I had a new lease on life, a second chance, and so I vowed to start exercising more and eating healthier, both of which I hadn't been doing.

Throughout high school, I was involved in numerous athletics (football, basketball, track, and wrestling). As a sophomore, to get stronger, bigger, and faster for football, I started weight training. To my surprise, and having never really enjoyed doing push-ups and pull-ups as a youngster, I fell in love with this new-to-me form of exercise almost immediately.

As keen as I was on getting stronger and putting on more muscle mass (which did happen), the thing that was most satisfying to me was the euphoria that followed each session. The natural high that lasted for hours on end was addictive - but in a good way. It was and still is empowering.

Results of the weight training carried over into the classroom (improved focus and memory), in sports (increased strength, size, and speed), in public (more confidence and self-awareness), and at home (better communication and sleep). With all of these health benefits, I continued to make lifting weights a priority four-to-five days a week, even through college.

At one point, though, to my dismay, I stopped enjoying the very thing that I had grown to love. My body had adapted to the program after a few years, and I wasn't making any progress in strength, size, or muscle tone. Frustrated and confused, I started experimenting with different training methodologies that I had studied.

In the early 1990s, I started following a protocol that was based on varying the number of sets, repetitions, and rest time for every workout, rather than changing them every few weeks, months, or even years, like most people did and still do. Although unusual, the program made a lot of sense to me. This unique method of training sparked a new energy in me, and the results were unlike anything I had experienced. My strength, stamina, and lean muscle mass all improved, and the workouts became challenging and fun again. I have continued to use this as the driving force for my clients and myself.

Bouts of insomnia, loss of employment, mild depression, failed relationships, and the passing of family, friends, and clients, have all challenged me throughout life. Through it all, regular exercise and proper nutrition are the two constants that have helped me deal with these obstacles.

Over the past three decades (1991 - present), I have lovingly worked as both a personal fitness trainer and weight management consultant. I have developed thousands of customized fitness and nutrition programs for a wide variety of clientele ranging in age from 12 to 92.

My programs have focused on a wide spectrum of goals: fat loss, strength, lean muscle mass, endurance, flexibility, speed, agility, balance, and stability. My clients have been middle-aged men and women, grandmas and grandpas, teenage boys and girls, amateur and professional athletes, couch potatoes and weekend warriors, and everything in between.

Many programs claim to work, but through my vast experience and extensive research, I feel I have developed programs that work better than most while being fun, challenging, efficient, safe, and effective. You can reach your goals by working smarter, not harder.

I've observed scores of folks in gyms throughout the country who perform weight training, stretches, foam rolling, cardiovascular exercises, and more, often incorrectly and unsafely. They have either been coached or trained wrong or not at all. Unfortunately, many follow advice from a magazine, friend, relative, or even a stranger at the gym touting bro-science.

I've also witnessed countless people in grocery stores, restaurants, sporting events, homes, and elsewhere, purchasing and consuming foods they think are healthy and safe to eat. The reality is that most individuals don't have a clue about nutrition because of all the myths, false marketing, and poor education about food.

It can be overwhelming for anyone to figure out what works and what doesn't when it comes to food and fitness. I have gained much insight into the many half-truths, fallacies, marketing ploys, and real facts dealing with exercise and nutrition, as well as other health related issues of clients. I feel compelled to share this knowledge and wisdom that I have acquired over the past three decades.

In the midst of all this, I hope to help you save time, energy, and money by debunking dozens of myths regarding food and fitness. More importantly, I aim to provide you with a sustainable and structured eating plan and training regimen that are both proven to be very effective and based in fact.

Human beings are designed to be active, eat properly, and get adequate rest. Poor health happens when we alter this equation. As much as I enjoy helping individuals balance these three pillars of health, I feel it's time to reach and teach a more extensive audience. With the current state of dismal health in this country, I feel a great sense of urgency to get this information out to the public.

According to the National Health and Nutrition Examination Survey (NHANES), in 2013-2014, two in three adults are overweight or obese; one in three adults are obese; one in 13 adults are extremely obese; one in six young people between the ages two to 19 are obese. These numbers are alarming!

Within the past few years, between raising a family, running a gym, training clients, speaking publicly, coaching kids, playing music, and enjoying the great outdoors, I've somehow managed to squeeze a few hours per week dedicated to writing this book. I believe much of the information within these pages is vital for every man, woman, and child. I hope you will find the broad selection of material surprising, enlightening, thought provoking, educational, motivational, inspirational, and even humorous.

Knowledge is power.

Enjoy!
Don Roberts

Acknowledgements

I am blessed, privileged, and honored to be in a career that affords me so much personal fulfillment. Every day at my fitness center, I feel a sense of camaraderie among members, trainers, and myself, all having a good time getting and staying in shape, as well as sharing stories or conversing about any current events or just telling jokes.

To see people strengthen physically and mentally before my eyes and to know that I played a role in that, however small or large, feels extremely rewarding.

The gym is really a "home away from home" for many folks, as well as me. Many of the gym members and clients have been a part of my world since the early 1990s. Several have been there for my father, mother, and friends passing; the birth of my two boys; my three bodybuilding contests, and so much more. A special bond has developed between me and these men and women, as they are really a second family.

Numerous people have been instrumental in my fitness journey and the writing of this book. It is appropriate that I give credit to these men and women who have helped pave my path.

- Teri Fithian Roberts (Durango District 9R P. E. teacher, graphic designer, horse trainer, my wife, and mother to our two boys) - who is always encouraging, knowledgeable, helpful, and has the patience of Job, despite the fact that I can be intense, moody, and demanding. Thanks, babe.

- Landon Roberts (oldest son) - who, through his discipline in lifting and nutrition, inspires me to stay healthy. After many years of writing this information in notebooks, he persuaded me to change my archaic ways and start typing in *Google Docs*.
- Kaleb Roberts (youngest son) - who, through his endless supply of energy, extraordinary willpower, and athletic abilities, keeps me young and uplifted.
- Don Roberts (Dad) - who taught me the values of the 4 D's (desire, dedication, determination, and discipline) as my guide to success in life, sports, and in fitness. Rest in peace, Pop.
- Lorraine Roberts (Mom) - who taught me that I could achieve anything that I set my sights on, if I worked hard enough for it. See you on the other side, Mom.
- Cynthia Roberts, Chris Roberts, Brian Roberts, Norman Roberts, Darlene Roberts Mellott, and Rosalyn Roberts (Siblings) - who encouraged and inspired me to give 100% to whatever I do.
- Nana Naisbitt (writer, Fit 24/7 gym member, and president of Chalkboard, a college consultancy) - who provided incredible advice, support, encouragement, and honesty while diligently editing this book.
- Gym Members/Clients - whose faith and success in my programs, motivated me to keep going in a career that I truly love.

- School Teammates/Classmates - who were like brothers and sisters to me and were always sources of encouragement, laughter, and friendship. Through the sweat, tears, and even blood occasionally, our time together (some since we were toddlers), whether playing sports or in the classroom, will be cherished forever.
- David Padoven (friend, Flexers Gym owner in Durango, and lifting partner for 10-years) - who inspired and motivated me in lifting and business practices. He elevated my career by making me manager and head trainer at Flexers Gym.
- Tony Teets (friend, national powerlifting champion, lifting partner, co-worker) - whose work ethic, sense of humor, and determination, elevated me and countless others to "give it our all" in the gym and in life. Even in the midst of battling Parkinson's Disease, he never complained. Tony silently taught us to smile in the face of adversity until it surrenders. Rest in peace, my dear friend.
- Carl Miller (World and National Olympic Style Weightlifting Coach, Assistant Strength and Conditioning Coach for the San Francisco 49ers, Dallas Cowboys, and Chicago Bulls) - who trained me on new exercises and techniques for power and strength.
- John Parrillo (National Strength and Conditioning Coach) - who inspired me by designing lifting programs that were unique, challenging, effective, and fun.

- Dave Cox (friend and college lifting partner) - who inspired, motivated, and encouraged me to work hard and have fun, in and out of the weight room.
- Sai Neesh (Main Street Gym owner in Durango) - who gave me my first job as a personal trainer back in 1991.
- Jean Rosenbaum M.D. (author, Main Street Gym member) - who initially motivated me to start writing a book long ago.
- Chad Midkiff (friend, lifting partner, bodybuilding competitor) - who provided much encouragement and laughter in and out of the gym for years.
- Steve Thyfault (Durango High School Football and Track & Field Coach) - who entrusted me to develop lifting programs and eating plans for his Four Corners Football Camps.
- Colleen Dean (Del Norte High School Track Coach) - who first taught me the value of plyometrics, as well as the value of rest after lifting weights.
- Eric McCrae (Del Norte High School Football Coach) - who motivated and encouraged me to start lifting weights at a young age, to become a bigger, stronger, and faster athlete.

Endorsements

"*Wellness Toolbox* sums up almost three decades of Don's work and experience. If you're ready to fast forward past all the health and fitness drivel online, this book is a must read! We're lucky to have it!"

Shane Ellison, MS, best-selling author: *3 Worst Meds; Hidden Truth About Cholesterol Lowering Drugs; Over-the-Counter Natural Cures; Health Myths Exposed*

"Don's gym has been part of my personal medical care over the years, and I have sent hundreds of clients and friends his way as he is one of the few fitness gurus that GET IT on all levels and know there is so much more to health and wellness than just exercising away that large pizza and quart of beer."

Dr. Nasha Winters, ND, FABNO, LAC, L.Ac, Dipl.OM, international speaker, naturopathic and integrative oncologist, bestselling co-author with Jess Higgins Kelley: *The Metabolic Approach to Cancer*, two-time cancer survivor

"*Wellness Toolbox* is filled with accurate information from credible sources. The format is a unique and refreshing way to understand nutrition and fitness. There is a lot of misinformation out there and you help to dispel it. I will recommend this book to my friends and patients."

Dr. John Rothchild, DDS, FAGD, MAGD, DAAPM, NMD, IMD, IBDM

"Thank you for distilling the facts: eat well, rest well, train well and therefore be well. Best of all, you explain how to go about all of that without gimmicks. "*Wellness Toolbox* is a great resource for health and well-being."

Dr. Antoinette Nowakowski, DC, DABCO, diplomate in chiropractic orthopedics, diplomate in internal health and wellness, 3rd Place 1996 *Mid USA Women's Bodybuilding* Masters Division

"We have learned that the safest way to evaluate any information is to be certain that it comes from a trusted source. Don Roberts has spent his career as a personal coach and trainer committed to assisting people to develop the physical and dietary habits that will lead to healthy lives. *Wellness Toolbox* records the lessons that Don has learned from years of direct involvement with, and the follow-up of his clients. His advice is backed by his conscientious study and recording of what has worked and what has not."

Dr. William Plested III, MD, General Surgery Specialist

"*Wellness Toolbox* has such valuable information, presented in a clear and concise manner, that had it been around while I was still competing, I believe I would have been a better lifter and a stronger athlete."

Betsy Skibyak-Ojanen, 12-time consecutive ADFPA/USAPL National Powerlifting Champion; 7-time WDFPF World Powerlifting Champion; USAPL Women's Powerlifting Hall of Fame; retired Phoenix Fire Captain/Paramedic (24 years)

"Don believes in enlightening his readers from the multidimensional view of fitness and health. His writing style is knowledgeable, user friendly, autobiographical, and permeated with current research discoveries. I plan to have a copy of *Wellness Toolbox* placed in our Fort Lewis College Library."

Chuck Walker, Professor of Exercise Science (emeritus), Fort Lewis College, PhD-Physical Education, University of Utah (1972), Fort Lewis College Men's basketball coach ('72-'83), University of Nevada: football, basketball, track & field athlete ('56-'60)

"Don has done a tremendous job putting *Wellness Toolbox* together. His knowledge base is expansive, and he constantly strives to keep up to date with current research on the body, health, and exercise."

Judith Noteboom, PT, CLT, MCMT, CFMS

"Don Roberts keeps a keen eye on health issues. He treats his gym like a lab - constantly measuring and tuning his approach to wellness and helping clients better understand their bodies. *Wellness Toolbox* is a perfect series of discussions outlining his approach to health in this modern life. It's all about asking the right questions - which is what Don does."

Dr. Gareth Hammond, MD, Orthopedic Surgeon

"What I've come to appreciate and respect about Don is his passion and persistence to the 'whole' process in training. This includes using his knowledge of nutrition and exercise and combining both to ensure success for women and men of all ages in their quest for better health."

Steve Thyfault, retired Physical Education Teacher and High School Football Coach of 30+ years

Introduction

In our diligent pursuit of health, we seem to have lost some of our common sense. We tend to believe that we can out-exercise a poor diet. Even greater, we think we can do this while getting far less sleep than is required for proper brain and body functions. Many believe that the answer lies in a pill, powder, or potion that will magically transform their body and/or their mind. When did we start down this strange and slippery slope? How did we lose sight of the fact that our bodies do best with proper rest, adequate nutrition, and more movement?

When information that isn't proven (aka a "myth") is talked about over and over again through time, it can become a so called "fact." The familiar "fact" that dogs and cats are color blind is a myth. Both have much better color vision than once thought. The myth probably started because canines and felines see colors differently than humans. Another fallacy is that sharks don't get cancer. Scientists have reported tumors in dozens of different shark species. The myth was created by I. William Lane to sell shark cartilage as a cancer treatment. (*Journal of Cancer Research, LiveScience*). Nutrition information is no exception to this conundrum. There are dozens of false beliefs regarding foods that are labeled as "healthy" and foods that are known as "harmful." There are numerous myths about exercise as well. Many people are spending a lot of wasted time on bogus exercises.

Throughout this book, I will expose many common myths about both nutrition and fitness. I hope to allay any misconceptions that you might have from past experiences and hearsay, so that you can make better choices about your own wellness based on the latest research and verified best practices. I intend to show how proper nutrition and exercise help you mentally, physically, and emotionally.

In order to cover a broad selection of material, while providing both factual and anecdotal data, I will debunk myths and facts in a concise fashion, with each subject covered in a few pages or less.

I will share testimonies and transformation photos of men and women of all sizes, ages, shapes, and abilities. As they say, a picture is worth a thousand words. It's incredible what the body and mind are capable of achieving.

In the span of my weight training career (since 1991), I have witnessed and been part of some pretty interesting happenings, in and around the gym. I will share several short stories with you as well. Some of these deal with unfortunate accidents, while others involve strange behaviors, dangerous situations, and funny occurrences.

My goal is to empower you to reach your full potential, both physically and mentally, by leading a vibrant, healthier and happier life. My hope is that you then spread the knowledge in your new wellness toolbox to your family, friends, neighbors, coworkers, classmates, and others.

Health is wealth. Don't just spend time, invest it in health!

Those who think they have not time for exercise
will sooner or later have to find time for illness."

~ Lord Edward Stanley,
British statesman 1851-1869

Section One

Fitness Myths and Facts

Physical activity, not drugs, is our best defense against everything from mood disorders to Alzheimer's disease to ADHD to addiction.

Fact.

Aerobic exercise physically remodels our brains for peak performance. Our culture treats the body and mind as separate entities, but they are not. Moving our muscles produces proteins that travel through our bloodstream and into the brain, where they play pivotal roles in the mechanism of our thought process. A Harvard Medical School experiment showed that voluntary exercise is better than forced exercise.

A 2000 Duke University Study shows that exercise is more effective at treating depression than the drug Zoloft. If exercise came in pill form, it would be advertised and sold everywhere, but companies can't patent exercise! Thus, pharmaceutical companies ignore exercise as a treatment and focus only on profitable drug treatments. Exercise is shown to improve symptoms of all these debilitating diseases: Alzheimer's disease, obesity, and bipolar disorders.

Naperville, Illinois students may be the fittest in the nation. Only 3% of sophomores are overweight. The national average is 30%. These students are also some of the smartest in the nation. In 1999, the eighth graders were among 230,000 students from around the world who took international standards tests. TIMSS (Trends in International Mathematics and Science Study) is usually dominated by students in China, Japan, and Singapore. The Illinois students finished sixth in math and first in science!

This success spurred the idea for the 2008 book, *Spark,* by John J. Ratey. The book demonstrates that learning at school is improved dramatically when students exercise early in the morning before their studies begin.

Neuroscientists discovered that exercise creates an unparalleled stimulus for the brain, making students ready, willing, and able to learn. I personally noticed a huge difference in my own focus, memory, and drive when I exercised first thing in the morning during high school and college. I continue this practice now, especially if preparing for a speaking engagement.

Aerobic exercise has a dramatic effect on neuromuscular systems that may be out of balance. Aerobic exercise is an indispensable tool for anyone wanting to reach his or her full potential. The results are a better mood, better reading skills, better sleep, and better math and science skills.

Called "Zero Hour," this unique approach to physical education has gained national attention and is now a model for gym classes throughout the world. These classes focus more on fitness than on sports. The philosophy is a that if PE classes can teach kids how to monitor and maintain their own health and fitness, they will learn lessons to serve them for life. Healthy habits, skills, and a sense of fun keep the kids hooked on moving, instead of habitually sitting in front of a TV or computer.

Statistics show that kids who exercise are likely to do the same as adults. Exercise for children leads to a heightened sense of focus and mood, less fidgeting in class, increased motivation, and invigorated feelings. This is the same for adults who are in the classroom of life.

Our brains are more like clay then ceramic, an adaptable organ much like a muscle. The more you use it, the stronger and more flexible it becomes. But erroneously, for many years, people thought that the best brain training was done through studying, reading, and problem solving. However, recent studies using brain imaging show that exercise stimulates the brain significantly more than solving a crossword puzzle or engaging in any "brain training" games.

Sustained aerobic exercise increases the birth of new neurons (neurogenesis). Exercise actually makes the brain bigger. Brant Cortright, PhD, professor of psychology at San Francisco's California Institute of Integral Studies, has shown that we can renew the brain at any age. The brain keeps growing throughout life, but rates of neurogenesis vary widely from person to person. Our quality of life is directly proportional to our rate of neurogenesis. We can increase the rate of neurogenesis at any age.

Another study by Scott Small, MD and Columbia University Professor of Neurology, shows that a three-month exercise regimen increased capillary volume in the memory area of the hippocampus by 30%. Increased capillary volume equals a greater memory. The hippocampus is essential to all four-levels of our humanness: body, heart, mind, and spirit. It is involved in physical movement (exercise and spatial learning of the body), mood and emotion (stress, anxiety, fear, and depression), cognitive (learning and new memory formation), and spiritual practices (mindfulness, devotion, and compassion). The hippocampus is the master key involved in all essential dimensions of human consciousness, and it is the ideal producer of new brain cells for brain self-renewal.

Standard recommendations advise half an hour of moderate physical exercise most days of the week, or 150 minutes per week. If that seems like a daunting task, start with just a few minutes per day and increase by 5-10 minutes per week until your goal is reached.

"Exercise is the single most powerful tool we have to optimize brain function. Exercise has a profound impact on cognitive abilities and mental health. Exercise is simply one of the best treatments we have for most psychiatric problems."

~ John J. Ratey, associate clinical professor of psychiatry at Harvard Medical School

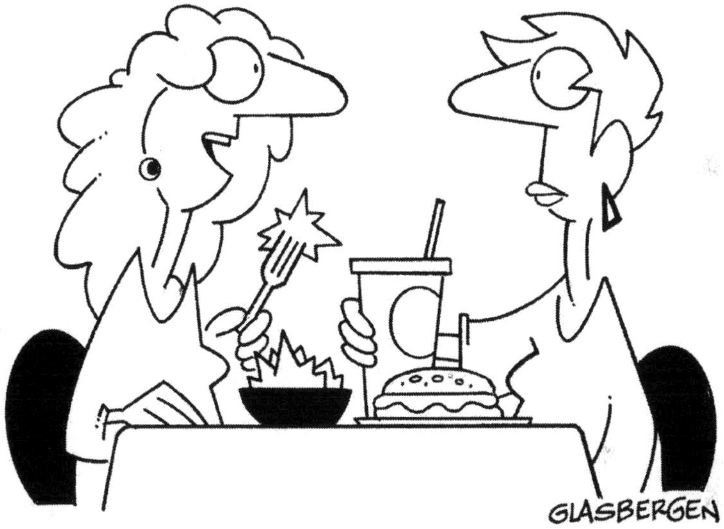

"I started working out and lost 6 inches from my waist, 4 inches from my hips and added 3 inches to my smile!"

A Don Story: Humble Beginnings

The bell rang loudly, as it always did. It was the last one of the day. Glad to be done with school, my sight was now set on physical activity, lifting weights in particular. Then a sophomore at Del Norte High School in South Central Colorado, weight training had become a major motivator for me. With brain chemicals (dopamine) and male hormones (testosterone and human growth hormone) surging through my veins, I had already begun a physical and mental transformation because of the past several months of lifting. My goal was to become bigger, stronger, and faster for football season the next year. The mental euphoria and stress relief were added benefits I hadn't expected, but gladly accepted.

As I entered the once dilapidated, now refurbished, old building, I was somewhat surprised that I was alone. "My teammates will be here in a few minutes," I presumed. This place was electrifying. Painted in our school colors of orange and black with mirrors mounted to the walls, my heart was filled with school pride. It was an exciting time to be a Del Norte Tiger. This little school in a town of roughly 1,500 residents had never had a weight room, only a couple of old machines that sat in the corner of the lobby in the basketball gymnasium, until a few parents and coaches got together and made it happen.

It was my upper body day, and I would be starting with the barbell flat bench press. Laying down with my back against the cool vinyl padding with my feet planted firmly on the floor, I tightly gripped the rough bar. My energy was high and the weight felt normal, if not a little easier than usual. I proceeded to add more weight. I was now into what is known in the lifting world as "working sets."

Primed and focused, I was ready for a personal best. The five-sets of five-reps program by Olympic weightlifter and strength building guru, Bill Starr, was the norm at the time, and this is what I had been following. That day, however, I wanted to change things up and try something new. I decided I would do eight-reps instead of five. Adding more Olympic plates to each side, the bar now totaled 135 pounds. Then I needed to add the safety collars. At five pounds each, they looked more like something out of a gladiator movie than a weight room. With protruding spikes of iron around the circumference, wing nuts at each hemisphere and leather cups on the internal chamber for grip, these old-style collars were bomb proof, unlike the plastic ones used by many facilities today. With the collars added, the bar was now at 145 pounds. This wasn't an unusual weight for me, I could easily do five-sets of five with it.

Still alone in the iron den, I laid back down and visualized doing eight-reps. I was motivated! Five-reps came relatively easy, then it was the 6th, but the 7th was tough. One more and I had my goal. I felt confident in the 8th. I made it half way back up and started to fatigue. "Suck it up Roberts!" I said to myself. "Push it or eat it!" echoed in my thoughts. It wasn't going any higher. Bringing the bar back down to my chest, I figured a little rest may help propel the 8th and final rep to the top, where it would be re-racked. I pushed again with all I could muster. It was not to be. I was pinned under the bar.

Akin to something out of a B-rated movie or maybe a cartoon, I was a teenager stuck under nearly 150 pounds of iron. "Help!" I shouted. After a few seconds I repeated my yell. Once more, my cry for help was not heard. I was still alone and helpless. I had to find a way to get this off my chest, and fast!

Guiding the bar toward my head was not an option or it could be trapped on my throat, and I'd possibly suffocate. I had to roll it down my abdominal wall and onto my thighs and try to force it off. For a grown man, this would probably not be such an ordeal, but for a 15-year-old it was a bit daunting.

With God as my copilot, I said a little prayer. I forced it down the remainder of my chest, onto my sternum, onto my abs, then onto my thighs. With the last ounce of strength I could muster, I sat up and gave the weight a final heave from my legs and onto the floor. With a loud crash, the weight was finally off of me.

What seemed like ten-minutes, probably took only one. Dazed, confused, and embarrassed, but thankful I was safe and had learned a valuable lesson. After resting for several minutes and gathering my senses, a few of my teammates had shown up. "Boy, could I have used you guys ten minutes ago," I exclaimed.

I had a lot to learn about weight training, but I knew it would always be an integral part of my life. I also learned that weight training alone carries risks. In addition to training with a reasonable amount of weight, it's important to have a spotter when attempting lifts that you are not sure of.

"Focus on a lifestyle that will last forever." ~ **Unknown**

Kids shouldn't start lifting weights until they're at least 12 years old.

Myth.

The current belief is that lifting weights is dangerous for the development of a child's growth plates. If proper exercise execution is performed, this is simply not accurate. In reality, kids naturally start lifting when they are toddlers. They do body squats, push-ups, deadlifts, and more, as soon as they are able to walk.

Weight training for kids improves sports performance, increases muscle mass and endurance, burns body fat, and improves bone strength. These are all beneficial for kids, whether they are athletes or not.

There's a great need for weight training with the rigors of football, basketball, hockey, soccer, baseball, and more. These sports place far more strain on the structures of kids than a well-executed lifting program.

Sports scientist, Dr. Mel Siff states in his book, *Facts and Fallacies of Fitness,* "The stresses imposed on the body by common sporting activities such as running, jumping, and hitting generate as much as 300% more impact than those imposed by powerlifting or Olympic lifting." European countries, as well as others across the globe, start kids lifting at an early age.

In North America, we tend to believe that machines are a much safer alternative for kids than free weights. Because of the static nature of a machine and their fixed pathways (which decrease our need to stabilize with our core), weight machines are inferior to free weights. Our bodies are not designed to perform static motion on fixed pathways. Machines appear safer to the uneducated eye, especially compared to Olympic lifts. Without a qualified coach or instructor, Olympic lifts can be dangerous. North American research has never proved, only assumed, that Olympic lifting and powerlifting are dangerous. Bone scans of children doing competitive lifting show significantly larger bone density with controlled, progressive lifting. Because of the dynamic nature of Olympic lifts, they are ideal for aiding in the development and coordination of movement skill for children. The essence of strength training is found in basic activities as running, jumping, and throwing.

Kids eight-to-ten-years-old are best suited to start learning form and function of basic lifts. Starting with a light bar or broom handle is best to perfect form. Kids should be taught the basics of set-up and movement and then produce the lifts minimal times per set. This method aids in developing quality motor sequencing and doesn't afford the opportunity of developing poor lifting habits during multiple repetitions and sets.

According to Teri M. McCambridge, a pediatric sports medicine specialist and chair of the American Academy of Pediatrics (AAP), weight training improves strength in teens and preteens. A child may start lifting weights as early as seven or eight years old. This is when balance and posture control are adequate, according to the AAP. McCambridge and colleagues wrote the AAP's 2008 policy statement on strength training for children and teens.

I started my boys, Landon and Kaleb, lifting weights at twelve years old. They have made vast improvements in strength, speed, agility, and lean muscle mass. I only wish I had started them a few years sooner. Supervision is crucial, especially with younger kids. Make sure the child's workouts are supervised by a qualified trainer or coach who emphasizes safety and correct technique above everything else.

"You are born weak and you die weak.
What you do in between is up to you."
~ Unknown

Crunches and sit-ups isolate the abdominal muscles and give you the best chance of developing a lean midsection and six pack.

Myth.

Even though these exercises hit parts of our core muscular structure, they can wreak havoc on our neck and lower back. Our core, which includes some 29 muscles, is designed to stabilize our spine more than mobilize it. Exercises like planks, bridges, side planks, dead bug, band torso twists, and prone cobra, just to name a few, are far superior to crunches and sit-ups, which only work a fraction (six-to-seven muscles) of the core.

Remember that you cannot spot reduce body fat on any area of your body, with the exception of liposuction, which I don't endorse. If you want to have good looking abdominal muscles, pay more attention to your diet. Eighty-percent of a "six-pack" has to do with food. More on that in the nutrition section of the book.

Core muscles act as an isometric or dynamic stabilizer for movement that transfers force from one extremity to another. Our core includes everything apart from our arms, legs and head, even our neck. Our core is incorporated in almost every movement of the body. Muscles of the core work together to bend your body, twist, move side-to-side, and stretch backwards and forwards.

A strong core provides better strength gains overall, as well as more effective movement. Our core really is the "powerhouse" of the entire body. The core muscles provide stability and strength for everyday living, as well as enhancing performance for sports and weight training. Having strong core muscles also reduces our risk of injury. Research shows that athletes with higher core stability have a lower risk of injury.

However, be careful because lifting weights too heavy or too fast can strain the pelvic floor muscles (an integral part of the core). Make sure you increase the weight slowly with good technique, engaging the core and inhaling and exhaling when weight training.

Weak glute (butt) muscles can cause overgripping of the pelvic floor muscles (PFM), pulling the sacrum out of alignment. Doing floor bridges and Kegel exercises help to balance this. Strengthening the PFM - a hammock like set of flat, sheet-like muscles and connective tissue that run from the pubic bone to the base of the spine and lie under the pelvis - mitigate erectile dysfunction and reduce incontinence.

Kegel (pelvic floor) exercises, which consist of repeatedly contracting and relaxing the muscles used to stop the flow of urine, are often done to strengthen the pelvic floor and help support our posture. Doing squats with Kegel exercises can help lengthen overly tight PFM. For proper muscle engagement and alignment, try to keep your knees stacked over your ankles and your pelvis untucked.

Lack of a natural lumbar (lower back) curve can be a sign of weak PFM, perhaps caused by too much sitting. As well, hunching (severe thoracic kyphosis) can lead to a weak pelvic floor. Doing a baby cobra move (gentle backbend face down on the floor) can help reverse rounding of the spine. Laying the upper back on a foam roller may also help.

This doesn't mean that you should never do isolation movements. Just make sure that you are prioritizing the more effective, integrative movements (planks, bridges, dying bug, mountain climbers, hanging knee ups, etc.) over the isolation movements (crunches, sit-ups, etc.).

"The best ab exercise is five sets of stop eating so much crap."
~ Unknown

Cardiovascular exercise is the best way to lose body fat.

Myth.

While cardiovascular exercise works our heart and lungs, burns some body fat, and increases our metabolism for a few hours, weight-bearing exercises burn more body fat. Cardio will burn calories, and the scale will probably show a lower weight; however, fat is not the only thing that burns, there are other tissues that could be compromised.

The more muscle you have, the more fuel you are constantly burning. A cardio machine is often seen as the quick fix for dropping body fat - and they are definitely useful if your goal is to improve cardiovascular health or endurance - but strength training is a powerful ally.

In a Penn State study, dieters lost 21-pounds whether they performed cardio or strength training. For the cardio group, six of those pounds were from muscle, while the lifters lost almost all fat and probably fit into their clothes better because of it. For every three-pounds of muscle that you gain, you can burn an extra 120-calories a day at rest.

Cardio is not necessary for fat loss. The maintenance of muscle tissue is what really matters. Lifting weights, especially large multi-joint motions like squats, deadlifts, lunges, rows, lat pulls, chest presses, shoulder presses, etc., increases our metabolism for a longer period of time than cardio exercises (up to 48-hours).

Performed as a circuit, or partnered with cardio, weight-bearing exercises are just as effective at working our heart and lungs as cardio, and weight bearing exercises build bone mass as an additional benefit. That doesn't mean you should stop doing cardio. It is one of the best ways to battle stress, which is a problem in and of itself when it comes to gaining unwanted fat. The best solution is a program that combines both cardio and strength training.

My favorite ways to get cardiovascular exercise in the gym are: airdyne bike, rower, elliptical trainer, and Jacob's Ladder. Using mostly my body, I like to do jump rope, sprints, or box jumps (when my knees can handle them). I either do a 15-to-20-minute interval or a 45-minute steady state version.

Be mindful that the calorie count on cardio machines is bogus. It is mostly a marketing ploy by the company who developed the machine. The actual number of calories being burned is determined by your weight, gender, age, muscle mass, and more. But don't get caught-up in caloric burn. You will continue to burn calories at rest after exercising.

"Strength training is a critical component of any program that emphasizes long-term fat loss."
~ Alwyn Cosgrove, fitness expert and author

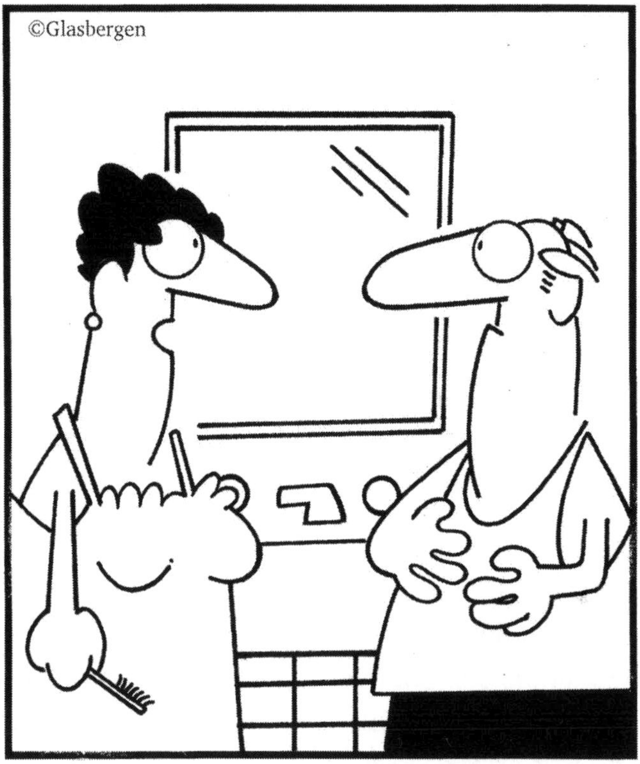

"Chasing the ice cream truck does not count as a summer fitness program."

Women and men should do the same exercises when it comes to weight training.

Fact.

One of the biggest misconceptions in the fitness industry is that men and women should train differently. Outdated ideas suggest that women shouldn't lift weights or train like men because they will build man-sized physiques and lose their femininity. Fueled by the media, as well as the fitness industry, this misconception helps sell gym memberships, as well as gender targeted activities. This is really a sexist movement that prevents women from realizing their true potential in fitness and health.

We all know the main differences between men and women. On average, women are smaller and have higher pitched voices. Adult women tend to have a higher proportion of fat and a lower proportion of muscle mass than men. Women also have slower metabolic rates, smaller lungs and hearts relative to body size, narrower shoulders, and shorter legs. However, muscles in men and women are essentially the same.

It's more an issue of attitude, culture, and tradition, than medicine or science. While the idea of strong, muscled women whose capabilities exceed those of many males may be odious to some people, there is no physiological reason why women should not participate successfully in weight training activities.

For decades, women have trained differently than men out of fear of getting bulky and looking like a guy. Women don't have the testosterone and growth hormone of men. Even with active testosterone hormones, building muscle can be difficult for a man.

By doing the big lifts like squats, lunges, deadlifts, rows, and chest presses, women will recruit much more muscle tissue and burn more fat. This will make women strong and lean. Women often mistake a muscle pump (the swelling of the muscle tissue) for muscle growth, but a muscle pump is short-lived and only last 90 minutes or so.

Many women believe that lifting heavy weights will bulk them up. Lifting heavy weights can actually slim you down. Women who lift a challenging weight for eight-reps burn almost twice as many calories as women who do 15-reps with lighter weights, according to a study published in *Medicine & Science in Sports & Exercise.*

I have been training women and men on similar programs for nearly thirty years. More than half of my success stories are from women who lift like men. Remember ladies, if you want to look like Jane, you've got to train like Tarzan!

"Strong is the new skinny." ~ **Unknown**

Lifting free weights is safer and more effective than using weight machines.

Fact.

Which is better: free weights or weight machines? Both free weights and weight machines are effective tools for achieving results. Free weights refer mostly to barbells, dumbbells, and kettlebells. Weight machines refer to weight stacks with pins, cables, and pulleys. Both free weights and machine weights do a good job of recruiting major muscles. While weight machines can sometimes be easier to use and tend to be less intimidating, they actually recruit less muscle tissue than free weights.

A study from Illinois State University showed that a free weight barbell bench press recruited 50-percent more muscle than the bench press machine did on the anterior deltoid muscle and 33-percent more on the medial deltoid. Pec and tricep recruitment were basically the same. This study shows that the stabilizing muscles of the shoulder are more active during the barbell bench press compared with the machine bench press. Using dumbbells for a bench press provides even more muscle recruitment than a barbell does.

Weight machines can be great at working the major muscles, but fall short for recruiting stabilizing muscles. Bench press machines, leg presses, leg extensions, leg curls, preacher curls, and Smith squats, just to name a few, are one-dimensional and lock your body into unnatural positions that compromise the integrity of the joints that are being used. They do not mimic any real-life movements like a free weight deadlift or a squat, for example.

"After mastering appropriate movement at some level, we next turn to load. There are many tools for load, including (but not limited to) barbells, kettlebells, dumbbells, rocks, bricks, but remember: correct and appropriate movement first," stated Dan John, world renowned strength coach.

According to Alwyn Cosgrove, world renowned strength and conditioning specialist, free weight squats activate 43-percent more muscle tissue than Smith machine squats. The dynamic nature of free weights is a better fit for athletic performance. Free weights are three dimensional, meaning you can work in three planes of motion: forward and backward, up and down, and side-to-side. This is how the body moves in normal daily activities.

Whether in a game or at practice, an athlete rarely moves their body in a single plane of motion. They are constantly running, jumping, stopping, starting, pushing, pulling, bending, and turning in various speeds, directions, and angles.

Free weights are also safer in most circumstances since they provide more freedom of movement. A machine locks you into a particular pattern that can pose a problem if you have a weight problem, an injury, or other limitation which does not allow for a precise movement.

However, free weights don't *always* provide the best or safest alternative. Because of limitations with an ankle or hip injury, for example, some people may be too uncomfortable doing a barbell deadlift and would be better suited for a cable deadlift.

To help you attain your goals and understand how the body moves and what you're trying to accomplish, contact a personal trainer or strength coach to help you design a program that fits your needs. A fitness professional can provide a safe, effective, and efficient program whether you are a couch potato, a weekend warrior, or a professional athlete.

"Focus on the pounds you lift, not on the pounds you weigh."
~ Unknown

A Don Story: Weight Machine Mishap

Tossing dirty towels into the gym washing machine, I heard a loud crash followed by an agonizing yell coming from the main floor. Rushing out of the tiny utility room, I scanned the gym for the source of the male scream. An older gentleman named John was pinned under a hack-squat machine (a large and heavy piece used for lower body weight training).

As I approached, I feared that he had broken both his legs. Rather than facing away from the upright padded back support, with feet braced on the metal platform below, he chose to do something I have never witnessed before nor since. He had stepped into the gap between the pad and the platform and proceeded to lift the safety handles without thought of what could happen. John was an interesting fellow, and let's just say that he was known to be under-the-influence of Lord-knows-what on more than one occasion while working out. Lifting and releasing the safety handles, he was holding well over a hundred pounds. Not able to sustain such a feat in the position he was in, the weighted sled (upper part of the machine) fell from about three-feet high and slammed him onto the floor.

I quickly grabbed the support handles and hoisted the weight off of him and back into its proper position. From the look on his face and the sight of his legs, it was apparent to me that he was injured. To what degree, I had no idea. With the sheer force of that much weight, he was lucky both of his legs weren't completely crushed. After I mentioned the possible need for an ambulance or paramedic, he gruffly said he could stand. I couldn't believe he didn't want medical attention.

Apprehensive, I helped him up. I stood in amazement of what had just happened. This man's lower limbs had just been slammed against a metal platform with over a hundred pounds. I'm not sure what was more shocking: the unorthodox way that he had gotten into the weight machine or that he had no apparent injuries.

Grabbing a first aid kit, we started dressing his wounds. Both of his shins were cut open and bleeding, but much less than I anticipated. Checking his vital signs and his body language, he appeared to be doing ok. First and foremost for his safety, but also to cover my ass, I repeatedly encouraged him to let me take him to the hospital for an examination. Being the stubborn, old, and grouchy codger that he was, I wasn't surprised when he denied every request. Astonished, I watched him get up after 10-minutes and continue with his work out.

Weight machines can be dangerous if you're not paying attention. Getting sound advice from a professional trainer before using weight machines can prevent an injury, as well as save you time and energy.

"Exercise and temperance can preserve something of our strength, even in old age."
~ Marcus Tullius Cicero, Roman statesman, orator, lawyer, and philosopher

High-intensity interval training (HIIT) has more benefits than traditional cardio.

Fact.

While steady-state cardio (continuous endurance) workouts certainly have their place in fitness, high intensity interval training (HIIT) gets it done faster with more benefits. HIIT workouts involve short bursts of intense exercise alternated with quick low-intensity recovery periods, typically lasting a total of 10-30 minutes. This popular form of training may be performed on all exercise modes, including rowing, cycling, elliptical training, weight training, stair climbing, walking, group exercise classes, swimming, and more.

HIIT workouts provide the same benefits as steady-state cardio, but in less time. HIIT training usually burns more calories than traditional workouts, especially afterwards. The excess post oxygen consumption (EPOC) period lasts for about two-hours after an exercise session. This is a period where the body is restoring itself to pre-exercise levels, and therefore using more energy. Because of these higher intensity workouts, the EPOC tends to be greater, adding 6-15% more caloric expenditure.

When designing your HIIT program, consider the frequency, intensity, and duration of the intervals, as well as the length of recovery intervals. The intensity should be equal to or greater than 80% of your estimated maximal heart rate (hard to very hard). With the talk test as a guide, having a conversation should be difficult. The intensity of the recovery interval should be 40-50% of your maximal heart rate. In other words, you should feel very comfortable before your next work interval.

Numerous studies show that different ratios of exercise to recovery improve both aerobic and anaerobic energy systems of the body. For example, a 1:1 ratio might be two-minutes of high intensity followed by two-minutes of low intensity. One example would be sprinting followed by walking. Another example would be rowing very fast followed by rowing slow. Another popular HIIT protocol is called the "sprint interval training method." This program uses 30-seconds of "all-out effort" followed by four minutes of recovery, repeated three-to-five times. The specific amount of time you exercise and recover should vary based on the activity you choose and the intensity of that exercise. During the high intensity efforts, the anaerobic system uses the energy stored in the muscles (glycogen).

One group of study participants did a two-minute warm-up on a stationary bicycle followed by a 20-second sprint, then rode slowly for two minutes. The group repeated that sequence two more times for a total of just 10 minutes. The other group rode steadily on the same bike for 45-minutes. After 12 weeks, both groups showed the same 20-percent increase in cardiovascular endurance.

In addition to weight training two-to-three times per week, I recommend HIIT training one-to-two times per week. I still perform steady state (moderate intensity) cardio for 30-45 minutes one-to-two times per week, as my right knee can't handle the high intensity like it used to. My personal favorite HIIT program is done on a Schwinn Airdyne bike that uses upper and lower body in an upright position. I like to do 20-30 second sprints followed by 20-30 second recovery. Repeated for six-to-eight times; this workout only takes 10-15 minutes. Remember, there are an almost endless array of choices that work for HIIT: rowing machine, elliptical trainer with arms, stepper, treadmill, jumping jacks, burpees, jumping rope, heavy-bag boxing, stair climbing, sprints, hiking, running, and more.

HIIT benefits include:

- Burning lots of calories in a short amount of time (up to 25-30% more in 30 minutes)
- A metabolic rate that is higher for hours after exercising
- Muscle gain (typically in the muscles being used)
- Loss of body fat and waist circumference
- Reduced heart rate and blood pressure
- Improved oxygen consumption
- Reduced blood sugar
- Mood enhancement

It is best to establish a base (foundational) level of fitness prior to starting a HIIT program. I recommend consistent aerobic training (three-to-four times per week for 20-60 minutes per session at a moderate intensity) for several weeks. This regimen produces muscular adaptations, improving oxygen transport to the muscles.

Sedentary people may have an increased risk of coronary disease if doing HIIT. Diabetes, hypertension, family history, cigarette smoking, and high cholesterol will increase this risk. Medical clearance from a physician may be needed before beginning a HIIT program.

"You will never know your limits until you push yourself to them." ~ **Unknown**

Functional training is fun, fast, and purposeful.

Fact.

It seems as though everyone is talking about functional training these days. Sometimes referred to as "developmental," "primal," or "sport specific," functional training uses exercises that allow individuals to perform daily activities more easily and without injuries.

"Function is, essentially purpose. When we use the word *function* we are saying that something has a purpose. So when we apply that term to training for sport we are talking about purposeful training for sports," states Mike Boyle, world renowned strength and conditioning coach.

However, functional training isn't just for sports, because purpose is at the base of everything we do. Whether changing a tire on a car, picking up a bag of groceries, pulling a hose across the yard, or chopping wood, functional training will help you perform these tasks with less effort.

The many benefits of functional training are:

- **Movement -** We are designed to be in motion, not sitting at a desk or on the couch. Functional training focuses on movement patterns, not on isolating individual muscles.
- **Fat burning -** By using full-body exercises that improve strength, endurance, and increase metabolism, functional training is a great fat burner.

- **Muscle density/tone** - Functional training develops lean, strong bodies by incorporating big movement patterns that recruit plenty of muscle tissue.
- **Core strength** - Functional training involves activities that target the core muscles of the lower back and abdomen, stabilizing the spine against external force through a variety of different body positions and movement patterns. These movements mimic the demand placed upon the body's core in everyday work and play.
- **Posture** - Functional training can help fix muscular imbalances and poor posture caused by our busy lifestyles, stressful jobs, and sitting in front of a computer.
- **Stability** - Workouts include stability, mobility, balance, flexibility, and strength training to keep your body constantly challenged in all areas of fitness.
- **Sports** - Improves the relationship between the nervous system and the musculoskeletal system, providing quick, reactive, and powerful movement patterns whether you are playing tennis, football, boxing, etc.

My recommended functional training exercises (in no particular order):

- Kettlebell clean-squat-press
- Kettlebell Turkish getup
- Kettlebell swings
- Kettle seesaws
- Kettle snatch
- Dumbbell suitcase squats

- Dumbbell walking lunges
- Dumbbell overhead press
- Dumbbell rows
- Dumbbell farmer carry
- Barbell squats
- Barbell deadlifts
- Barbell cleans
- Barbell push press
- Barbell landmine twist
- TRX elevated planks
- TRX pistol squats
- TRX rows
- TRX press
- Med-ball slam
- Deadmill
- Burpees
- Jacob's Ladder
- Push-ups
- Pull-ups
- Jumping rope
- Kickboxing
- Jumping jacks
- Seal jacks
- Slideboard
- Box jumps
- Sled push/pull
- Battle ropes
- Tire flip
- Planks
- Dying bug
- Band torso twist

- Cable torso twist
- Wall sit
- Rope climb

You get the best results in the weight room, on the court, track, mat, field, course, slopes, and more by incorporating a well-balanced mix of these functional movements.

I recommend doing a circuit of a few of these fabulous functional training exercises to achieve the most benefits and to prevent imbalances which tend to lead to injury.

In my opinion, functional training circuits are the ultimate form of HIIT, since they combine strength, mobility, stability, balance, agility, and cardio. I prefer doing each for 30-60 seconds followed by 30-60 seconds of rest. Performing the workout one-to-three times per week only takes 15-45 minutes. Change it up by selecting a different combination of exercises each time you train. I'll bet you will find a functional training circuit to be one of the most fun, most challenging, most efficient, and most effective workouts you've ever encountered!

As always, contact a professional trainer to provide proper instruction on these and other exercises.

"Think of your training as a vehicle
to improve performance, not just improve strength."
~ Mike Boyle, World renowned strength and conditioning coach

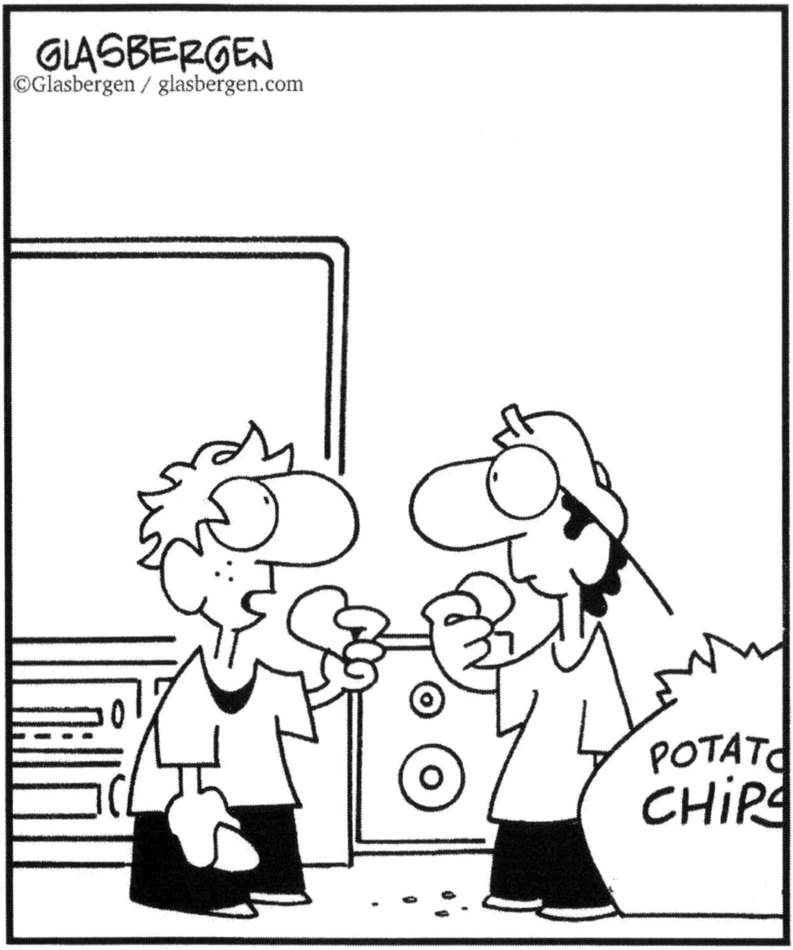

"They say kids these days are overweight because we don't get enough vigorous exercise. Maybe we should chew faster!"

Sweating is a sign of being out of shape.

Myth.

The average person has two-to-four million sweat glands. These vital glands are essential to human survival, cooling our body and protecting it from overheating. Athletes and others in shape tend to sweat more than other people because their bodies have become more efficient at keeping cool.

Sweating increases blood circulation in the body, boosts endorphins, detoxes the body, prevents colds and illnesses, lowers kidney stone risk, and even controls acne. The amount of sweat produced by an individual has to do with his or her fitness level, gender (men tend to sweat more), hydration, air temperature, and humidity.

Here are several myths about sweat:

- **Myth #1 - You can lose fat by sweating.** Any weight loss that might occur from sweating is simply water weight, which is instantly regained from drinking water.
- **Myth #2 - Not sweating means your workout wasn't intense enough.** The fact is your metabolic state, temperature of the room, and clothing fabric are all factors in how much you sweat.
- **Myth #3 - Only overweight people suffer from excessive sweating.** In truth, excessive sweating, or hyperhidrosis, is a medical condition that causes people to sweat 4-5 times more than

normal, affecting over 365 million people worldwide.

- **Myth # 4 - We only sweat on hot days.** The fact is the body is constantly adjusting to temperature by releasing moisture.
- **Myth #5 - Sweat causes acne.** Acne is actually caused by oil clogging your pores.
- **Myth #6 - Yellow stains on your clothes are caused by sweat.** Actually, oil and bacteria from your skin form yellow stains.
- **Myth #7 - Sweat causes body odor.** Perspiration odor is actually caused by bacteria.
- **Myth #8 - Men have more sweat glands than women.** Women actually have more sweat glands than men, but men's are more active.
- **Myth #9 - Underarms have the most sweat glands.** The fact is our feet have the most sweat glands, but since they are usually covered with sweat absorbing socks, we don't notice them sweating as much.

"Sweat is magic. Cover yourself in it daily to grant your wishes."
~ Unknown

It is not possible to be fat and fit.

Myth.

You can't judge a person's fitness by looks alone. Despite what the general population believes and what the media stories say, based on unpublished research, it is possible to be fat and fit. That overweight gal on the stationary bike may be healthier than the skinny guy sitting in his recliner.

The "fat but fit" contention has been going on for decades, and it will probably continue for decades more. However, the research shows that overweight people who exercise can absolutely be healthier than thin people who don't.

While extra body fat isn't recommended, exercise has positive impacts regardless of your weight. Those impacts are sometimes enough to offset the negative effects of being overweight. "What we're learning is that a body that exercises regularly is generally a healthy body whether that body is fat or thin," wrote Glenn Gaesser, PhD, a professor of exercise and wellness at Arizona State University and the author of *Big Fat Lies: The Truth About Your Weight and Your Health.*

A 2011 study showed that moderate exercise and a well-rounded diet changed the ways obese patients' bodies functioned and that "these lifestyle-induced adaptations occur independently of changes in body weight or body fat." Another study from 2014 found that "Physical activity has a protective effect on biomarkers in normal, overweight, and obese individuals, and overweight (not obese) active individuals have a similar cardiovascular profile than normal weight inactive individuals." A 2015 study showed that "only those individuals who were inactive were at a significantly increased risk of all-cause mortality independent of overweight/obesity status."

I've trained overweight football players, basketball players, skiers, bikers, weight lifters, swimmers, and more. These athletes were more fit than some of the thinner non-athletes I have worked with.

So while you may not be seeing the numbers changing on the scale or even with your clothes, know that what's happening on the inside is what really counts. Focus on fitness not fatness!

"Exercise to be fit, not skinny. Eat to nourish your body."
~ Unknown

BMI (body mass index) is a poor way to determine one's state of health.

Fact.

Simple to apply and noninvasive to perform, BMI is used countless times every day by health care providers, but it is a poor marker for overall health and well-being. BMI alone doesn't tell the whole story, far from it. It only uses weight and height to determine obesity or lack thereof. An adult with a BMI of 25 is considered overweight and 30 or higher is considered obese.

The person that dreamed up BMI said explicitly that it should not be used to indicate the level of fatness in an individual. A Belgian named Lambert Adolphe Jacques Quetelet introduced BMI in the early 19th century. He wasn't a physician, but rather a mathematician. He produced the formula to give a quick and easy way to measure the degree of obesity of the general population to assist the government in allocating resources. In other words, it is a flawed 200-year-old measurement still in use today.

The flaw is that it is based on bodyweight and not on body composition. BMI doesn't measure body fat. A person may lose fat and gain muscle and their BMI won't change a bit. We need to look at more factors like muscle mass, bone mass, and hydration versus just fat! An athlete with lots of muscle mass may be considered obese using BMI figures. Also, older folks who may have lost muscle could show deceptively low BMI. The CDCP (Centers for Disease Control and Prevention) thinks BMI is a reasonable indicator of body fat, but does not recommend it as a diagnostic tool. Alternate methods that should be considered are skinfold caliper tests, waist and hip measurements, and bioelectrical impedance.

We have used both skin calipers and measuring tapes here at my gym, Fit 24/7 since 2002. Men with a body fat of 26% or more are at risk, as are women with 32% or more. Men with a waist measuring 40 inches or more and women with a waist 35 inches or more are at high risk of developing obesity related diseases like high blood pressure, certain cancers, and diabetes.

How do you feel? How do you look? How do your clothes fit? How do you perform? These are the questions that I believe we should be asking, rather than, what is your BMI?

"No matter how slow you go, you are still lapping everyone on the couch." ~ **Unknown**

Full-body weight training workouts are better than split routines (one or two body parts worked per day) for strength and conditioning.

Fact.

Full body workouts are the way the old-timers lifted before bodybuilding and powerlifting drugs came onto the scene. Veteran bodybuilders Reg Park, Vince Gironda, Leroy Colbert, George Eiferman, and many more, trained with full-body methodology. They were very strong and had slabs of muscle from head to toe.

World renowned strength and conditioning coaches like Mike Boyle, Alwyn Cosgrove and Chad Waterbury, who have all been in the industry for 20+ years, prefer full-body training over split routines for better strength, increased muscle, and improved performance. Cosgroves states, "Body-part split workouts are shown to be the least effective for the masses and have more failure rates than any other methodology." Waterbury says "For decades most trainees worked out 3-days per-week on full-body programs with great success. Tens of thousands can't be wrong."

Full-body weight training workouts are superior because they:

- Burn more body fat
- Lower levels of boredom
- Lower time commitment
- Recruit more muscle tissue
- Provide useful (functional) movements

- Are fun, challenging, unique, and efficient
- Can be better for our nervous system and adrenal glands
- Are great for kids, beginners, adults, as well as advanced athletes
- Provide greater hormone release (testosterone and growth hormone)
- Allow muscle groups to be worked 2-3 times a week, not just once a week

Purposely choosing a day or two of rest after each full-body workout allows for optimal recovery for the muscles and prevents mental and physical burnout from exercising too often.

"Warning: Exercise has been known to cause health and happiness."
~ Unknown

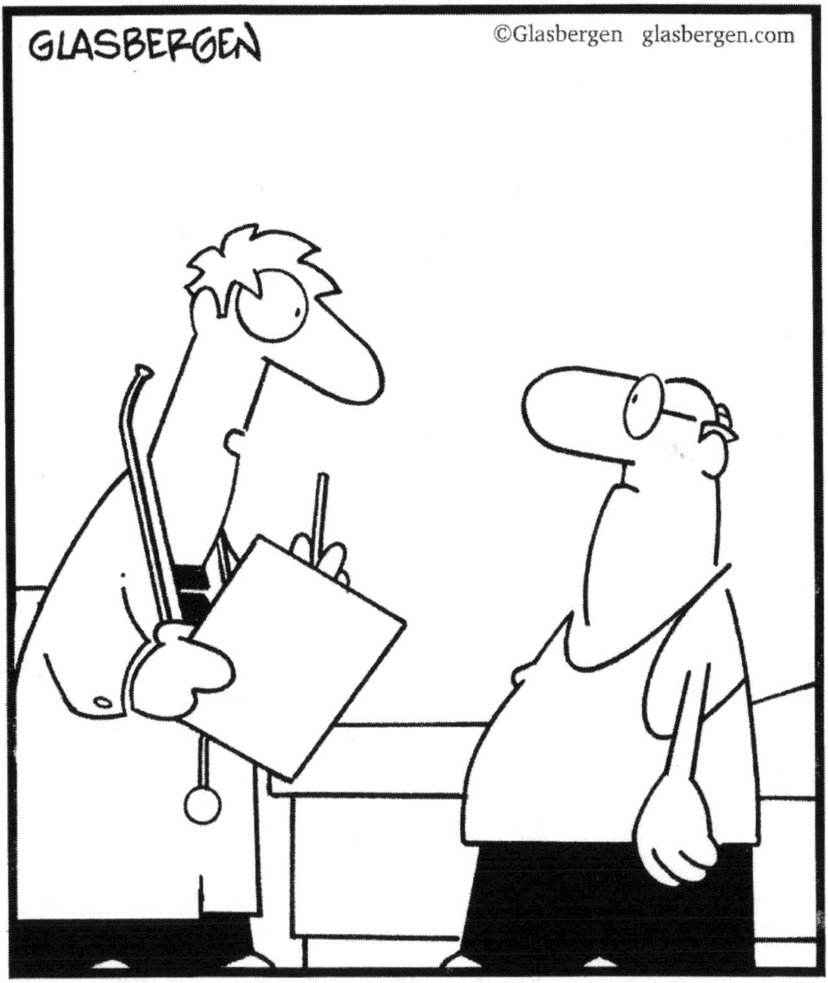

"What fits your busy schedule better, exercising one hour a day or being dead 24 hours a day?"

Deadlifts are just as effective as bicep curls and tricep extensions for arm strength and size.

Fact.

Considered by many to be the king of all exercises (some say squats), this incredible exercise works the lower and upper body like no other, creating a stronger, more muscular physique. If performed correctly, the deadlift will build unparalleled muscle throughout much of the body, while strengthening most of the major muscle groups.

Strength and hypertrophy (size) are systematic responses and effects, not localized ones. In other words, big compound movements, like deadlifts, work most of the body, rather than isolating specific body parts like bicep curls and tricep extensions.

Deadlifting will strengthen the entire back, making this lift ideal for rehabilitative and preventative purposes. The deadlift is actually the most effective exercise for building the core strength that supports all other muscle groups. Forcing the whole body to work, the deadlift works more muscles simultaneously than any other movement.

A 10-week study from Ball State University compared the effects of a weight training program on strength and arm circumference of men. They divided the subjects into two groups. Group 1 performed four compound upper-body exercises with deadlifts being a primary move. Group 2 used the same program as group one, but added bicep curls and tricep extensions. Both groups significantly increased strength and arm size. However, the addition of direct arm training for Group 1, with the curls and extensions, produced NO additional strength or arm circumference after 10 weeks, compared to Group 2!

In any workout that includes both deadlifts and squats, it is always best to do deadlifts after squats. Deadlifts require stabilization from the low back. Squats require perfect spinal alignment. Improper alignment may cause a strain in the lower back. Deadlifts strengthen the lower back, but also fatigue it; much more so than squats. If done intelligently, you can squat and deadlift on the same day. Some people prefer doing deadlifts with back exercises on the same day.

There are many styles of deadlifts: traditional, Sumo, Romanian, etc. The types of weights vary as well: barbell, hex bar, dumbbells, kettlebells, etc. One style and type may feel uncomfortable, while another may suit you well. Try a variety to see what fits your body structure and mechanics best. And always remember to never round your back.

"If weakness is the disease, deadlifts are the cure."
~ Unknown

Squats are complicated and dangerous, causing knee and back problems.

Myth.

Squats, as well as deadlifts, are amazing for overall fat loss, lean muscle gain, strength, and vertical jump.

This hip-dominant exercise that recruits over 200 muscles can be done with dumbbells, kettlebells, a barbell, a medicine ball, TRX straps, or the body only. The critical data on squatting has been misinterpreted, misunderstood, and ignored for decades.

Squats work muscles in the entire body and also create an anabolic environment promoting body wide muscle building. By increasing testosterone and growth hormones, squats help the whole body build muscle and lose fat. Functional exercises like squats make day-to-day activities easier.

Humans have been squatting since the hunter-gatherer days, promoting mobility and balance. Squatting is a natural movement. Squats help the body move more efficiently. They also help prevent injuries by strengthening the stabilizer muscles of the legs, hips, and core, as well as ligaments and connective tissue. Squatting also improves flexibility in the ankles and hips. Squats boost sports performance by improving jump height and speed.

Don't be afraid to squat past 90-degrees. This activates the leg muscles the most, compared to half squats. Full squats are not bad for the knees unless your technique is poor. As long as your spine is straight (from the top of the cervical vertebrates to the bottom of the sacrum) and you're not feeling pain in your knees, you should be fine. Foot placement and width has little to no effect on muscle activation. Contrary to popular belief, there is no observable difference in muscle activation between front (weight on the anterior side of the body) and back (weight on the posterior side of the body) squats.

Squatting is part of virtually every professional, collegiate, and high school athlete's training program. Squats tone your backside, abs, and entire body. Squatting also helps remove waste products from the body by pumping body fluids at the cellular level, which helps to deliver nutrients to all tissues, including organs and glands.

Since the age of 15, I have incorporated squats into my exercise routine. I can say with certainty that squats have been the best exercise for my athletic career, bodybuilding success, fat loss, muscle gain, and even cognitive function. Groundbreaking research, published in *Frontiers of Neuroscience* in March 2018, shows that neurological health depends as much upon signals sent by the body's large, leg muscles to the brain as it does on signals from the brain to the muscles.

A ten-years-long British study of 324 twins found that those with the most powerful legs showed the least decline in thinking skills. The more muscular and stronger twin performed roughly 18% better on memory and cognitive tests than the weaker twin. "I was quite surprised by the strength of the findings," said Dr. Claire Steves, a senior lecturer at King's College in London, "because to be honest, I am someone who has always in the past prioritized work of the mind over work of the body. This study brings home to me that the brain needs exercise to keep fit." She suspects that working muscles release biochemicals that travel to the brain and affect cellular health there.

Split squats (one leg behind the other) can be even more effective for performance, balance, and safety than traditional squats (legs side-by-side). Since we walk and run on one leg at a time, not two, give split squats a try!

Whether using a barbell, dumbbells, kettlebells, or just your body, the technique of your squat must be perfected to maximize performance and to avoid injury. Have a qualified and experienced fitness professional show you the proper technique of this incredible exercise.

"You won't get the butt you want by sitting on the one you have."
~ Unknown

A Don Story: Split Squats

A friend and coworker of mine, David, was built like a brick outhouse. At six feet tall and two-hundred plus pounds, he looked like a bodybuilder: broad shoulders, big ripped arms, and a narrow waist, albeit small to average thighs. One day at work, I asked him what gym he was a member of. He said he only trained at his house. One weekend afternoon he invited me over to lift weights.

Walking into his modest home, I noticed several pictures hanging in a hallway. Many were of his family, but one stood out. It was an action shot of him as a high school athlete playing football. After asking a few questions, I found out he was an All-State defensive end for a small town located in central Colorado, known to be a powerhouse in football for most of my childhood.

Down the hall was his weight room. Actually, it was a room with a few weights in it. It was certainly not what I expected. An Olympic flat barbell press, an EZ curl bar, and a rowing machine is all I remember. Spotting him while we did the bench press, I knew he was a bit stronger than I. Moving on to some EZ bar curls afterward, his strength showed through again. At 25 years old, he had a couple of years of lifting experience on me. I was only 23.

How do you train your legs? I asked. He responded that he did not. After realizing he wasn't joking, I showed him how to properly do squats and split squats with just a 45-pound bar. Legs were something I had always prioritized. He was more of an upper body guy.

Watching me work up to 135 pounds (a 45-pound plate on each side of the bar), he figured he'd give it a try. Having worked up to that weight for a few years, I was apprehensive about him trying such a feat. However, he was a grown man. If he wanted to attempt it, who was I to stop him. After he positioned it on his upper back, he was ready for his first rep. What happened next was like something from America's Funniest Videos.

He came down quickly, falling forward. The large Olympic plates crashed into the wall with a thunderous sound, knocking pictures off of the walls and onto the floor. In addition, there were now two large holes in the sheetrock. It was as if a demolition crew had come in and started with sledge hammers.

Fortunately, only his pride was hurt. Squats and split squats soon became part of his weekly training ritual, and they should be part of yours.

"Keep your squats low and your standards high."
~ Unknown

Running causes knee problems and arthritis.

Myth.

Running itself will not cause arthritis. However, if you already have arthritis, and no cartilage in your knee, and bone-on-bone contact, running will make it worse. Running actually helps future arthritic patients be more active in their later years. The motion helps bring more fluid to the knee and keeps them moving. The lighter you are and how well you land on your feet are important. Not everyone hits the ground with the same force. Heavier people will cause extra force on the knee joint.

According to Dr. Stephen G. Rice, Director of Sports Medicine at Jersey Shore University Medical Center, the person who is active and fit is defending best against arthritis. There's a happy medium between whether you run smart (slowly building up your endurance) and putting too much extra force on your knees. People who are genetically predisposed to arthritis, no matter how well they run, will end up developing arthritis anyway.

Chris Troyanos, certified athletic trainer and medical coordinator for the Boston Marathon, says that running is healthy and good for most people, but it's a matter of how you get started in running and whether you progress slowly, as recommended. When considering a running program, you might want to start with a walking program initially, then ease into an easy running program, before running a marathon, for example.

Dr. Michelle Wolcott, associate professor at the University of Colorado School of Medicine, states that if you haven't had an injury, like a torn ligament or a broken bone, which can predispose you to arthritis, then your chances of creating arthritis are minimal. Weight-bearing exercise, like running helps prevent osteoarthritis and osteoporosis. Repetitive motion and weight-bearing activities are good for the joints, and running does that.

A large study of almost 75,000 runners by Berkeley National Laboratory found "no evidence that running increases the risk of osteoarthritis, including participation in marathons." The runners in the study actually had less overall risk of developing arthritis than people who were less active.

There's absolutely no evidence that running alone causes osteoarthritis or arthritis. People who claim that running caused their knee problem likely already had a knee injury.

"Running is nothing more than a series of arguments between the part of your brain that wants to stop and the part that wants to keep going."

~ Unknown

After age 60, you cannot gain muscle mass or strength.

Myth.

With only a fraction of adults engaging in exercise, age related muscle mass loss (sarcopenia) affects roughly 45% of adults in the United States (53% of men and 43% of women). Physical inactivity can cause a loss of 3-5% of muscle mass after age 30. Most adult humans peak with muscle mass in their thirties and forties. However, you can rebuild aging muscles whether you are middle-aged or older.

"Our lab and others have shown repeatedly that older muscles will grow and strengthen," says Marcas Bamman, director of the UAB Center for Exercise Medicine at the University of Alabama at Birmingham. In his studies, men and women in their sixties and seventies who began supervised weight training developed muscles that were as large and strong as those of your average 40-year-old. The key is regular and progressive weight training. "If you don't belong to a gym, consider joining one," says Bamman. In order to initiate the biochemical processes that lead to larger and stronger muscles, you need to push your muscles until exhausted. Bamman recommends doing two-to-three sets of eight-to-twelve repetitions every other day (three-days per-week).

Sandy Palais (73 years old) of Tempe, Arizona, does weight training several days a week. She started lifting 10 years ago after being diagnosed with osteoporosis. Palais now competes in weightlifting for local Senior Olympics. Believe it or not, she has benched 80 pounds; squatted 135 pounds;

and deadlifted 165 pounds! All with free weights. It's no wonder she has a drawer full of gold and silver medals. Did I mention she is over 70?

Analysis of 39 studies shows that among 1,300 adults over the age of 50, muscle mass can be increased by an average of nearly 2.5 pounds in only five-months. Weight training not only reverses age-related muscle loss, it actually creates new muscle. Research shows that the greater the intensity of the weight training program, the greater the results. Adults who lifted the most weight increased their lower and upper body strength by almost one third.

In the decades that I have been training clients, many of them have been over 60 years old. Several members at my Fit 24/7 gym are lifting weights in their seventies and eighties. Consequently, I have seen incredible transformations in muscle strength, muscle size (hypertrophy), and muscle tone. Linda Allenbaugh, at 70 years old, increased her strength on the bench press 400% in eight-weeks (eight reps at 15 pounds to eight reps at 60 pounds).

"We don't stop playing because we grow old;
we grow old because we stop playing."
~ George Bernard Shaw, Irish playwright

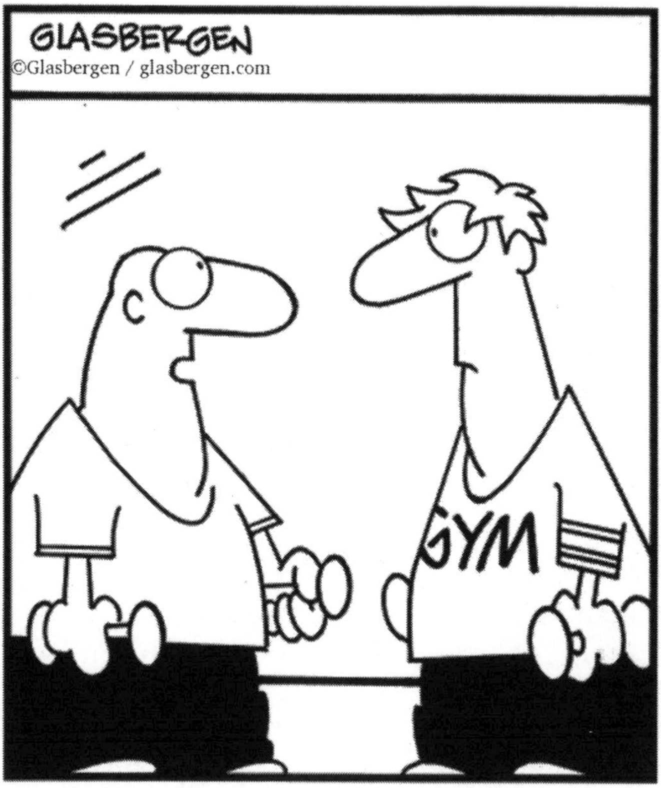

"My trainer says I should listen to my body. My wife says she's been listening to my body for years!"

We are all pre-programmed to live a certain number of years. Our genetics determine this. Exercise and nutrition have very little to do with it.

Myth.

According to Dr. Walter M. Bortz II, in his book *We Live too Short and Die too Young*, "humans were designed to live to 120 years." The absence of exercise shortens our life span. The fact of the matter is, exercise decreases (in a good way): resting heart rate, blood pressure, blood thickness, body fat, blood sugar, insulin levels, low density lipoprotein, depression, and memory loss. On the flipside, exercise increases (in a good way): heart pumping capacity, intestinal elimination, muscle mass and strength, metabolic rate, high density lipoprotein, and quality of sleep.

Dr. Bortz estimates that our biogenetic max life is 120 years, but most Americans die in late-middle age, around 76. Jeanne Calment, who died in 1997 at 122, lived longer than any person in recorded history. One-hundred-five-year-old Japanese woman named, Hidekichi Miyazaki, is still a competitive sprinter in the 100-meter dash. Ida Keeling of New York City didn't start running until her mid-sixties, but now at 100 years old, she is the reigning national champion in the 60-meter dash: 29.86 seconds. "You see so many older people just sitting around - well, that's not me," says Keeling. "Time marches on, but I keep going."

Toxins that we breathe, absorb, or eat, and wear and tear on the body are also to blame for our shortened life spans. If cause of damage can be removed or corrected, life expectancy could be extended. All organs and vital functions show a gradual reduction in capacity with time. No one has been proven to die of "old age." Most deaths are results of a sharply localized problem like hemorrhaging, blood clotting, or a strategically placed tumor.

Age is a very complex thing that involves many body systems. Changes occur in cells that alter the cell's ability to function or respond to external stress or infection. If abnormalities like disease, trauma, behavioral maladaptation, and self-destruction were controlled, we would all live much longer.

"We haven't found any biological reason not to live to 110," says Dr. Robert Butler, First Director of the National Institute on Aging. The improvements in life expectancy (from 45 to 76) in the last 75-years appears to be from improvements in medical care at birth, conquering many infectious diseases, the discovery of antibiotics, and better nutrition and hygiene. This dramatic lengthening of lifespan is predicted to continue. By 2050, 400,000 Americans will be 100 or older, according to the U.S. Census Bureau. And a recent cover of National Geographic Magazine showed a picture of a baby with the headline, "This Baby Will Live To Be 120."

The number of people living to 100 has increased 71% in the last decade and has spiked 500% since the 1980s. According to Global Agewatch Index, there are now more than half-a-million people aged 90 and above in the UK, and nearly 14,000 of them aged more than 100.

"How old would you be if you didn't know how old you are?"
~ Satchel Paige, Hall of Fame Major League baseball pitcher

Unless you are a competitive athlete, setting fitness/nutrition goals is basically a waste of time.

Myth.

Setting goals should be a part of your life, whether it's losing weight, exercising more, sleeping more, stressing less, etc. Experts say that selecting an objective is the best way to achieve a goal. Ask yourself, "What do I want to achieve?" and think seriously about the answer. The primary purpose of a goal is to guide you in creating the system you need to make the change.

Helpful strategies:

- **Give your goals a hierarchy (goal competition).** Focus on one goal at a time. Pick a dream so big, it will motivate you every day. You don't need more time, just decide! Think of a rosebush; cut away the good buds so the great ones can stand out. Consistently trim down and refine your goals.
- **Stack your goals.** You're two to three times more likely to accomplish your goals if you plan the when, where, and how. Examples might be: I will partake in 30-minutes of vigorous exercise on (day?) at (time?) at (place?)... after/before (current habit?). I will (new habit?)... Before I eat lunch I will go to the gym. Link new goals to something you're already doing.
- **Set boundaries.** Think about the minimum and maximum threshold: "I want to lose at least five

pounds this month." It would be even better to say, "I want to lose at least five pounds, but not more than 10." Setting an upper limit makes it easier to sustain progress without frustration or burnout. Setting lower limits prevents laziness. To achieve the goals consistently, you must have the right goal and the right system. Try to align your environment with your ambition. For example, if you keep water with you at work, you're less inclined to drink a soda. It's hard to stick to positive habits when you are in a negative environment. For example, it's hard to eat healthfully if junk food is in the kitchen.

According to data, the top two New Year's resolutions are to lose weight and to get fit. While these goals are admirable, they aren't specific enough. The American Council on Exercise (ACE) recommends using the SMART goal method as a strategy for effective goal setting.

According to this SMART method, goals should be:

- **Specific** - The goal must precisely state what is to be accomplished.
- **Measurable** - The goal must be quantifiable, so you know if you achieved it or not.
- **Attainable** - Don't make the goal too difficult.
- **Relevant** - The goal needs to relate to your personal needs and interests.
- **Time-bound** - Deadlines help keep you focused and on track.

Using the SMART method, you can change your goals so they're specific and easier to accomplish. Instead of saying,

"I'm going to lose weight," you could say, "I'm going to lose 15-pounds by April." I have used the SMART goal method with my clients for over 20 years with great success. It is the best and simplest method that I have found.

Schedule a personal training session with a fitness professional for next week while you're feeling motivated today. The human mind loves feedback. Use a fitness/nutrition journal to help you achieve your goals.

"Goal setting can be so powerful.
It provides focus. It shapes our dreams.
It gives us the ability to hone in on the exact actions
we need to do to get everything that we deserve in life."
~ Jim Rohn, American entrepreneur, author,
motivational speaker

Visualization techniques and practices can have a profound effect on achieving your goals.

Fact.

Picturing yourself succeeding in your mind before actually doing something in the real world can be extremely powerful.

In one study, scientists mapped the brains of weightlifters. They made a startling discovery. The same areas of the brain lit up when the weightlifters hoisted hundreds of pounds above their shoulders or merely imagined doing so! This research revealed that mental practices are nearly as effective as true physical practice. Doing both is the most effective.

In his study on everyday people, Guang Yue, an exercise psychologist from Cleveland Clinic Foundation in Ohio, compared "people who went to the gym with people who carried out virtual workouts in their heads." He discovered a 30% muscle increase in the group who went to the gym. Amazingly, the group of participants who did only mental exercises of the weight training still increased muscle strength by almost half as much (13.5%). This average remained for three months following the mental training.

The Soviets started using mental imagery back in the 1970s. Many famous athletes and celebrities have used this popular technique: Lindsey Vonn, Arnold Schwarzenegger, Muhammad Ali, Tiger Woods, Michael Jordan, Will Smith, Jim Carrey, Oprah Winfrey, and countless others.

Brain studies show that thoughts produce the same mental instructions as actions. Numerous cognitive processes of the brain are impacted by mental imagery: attention, perception, motor control, planning, and memory.

The brain is getting trained for performance during visualization - increasing self-confidence and self-efficacy, improving motor performance, priming the brain for success, and increasing states of flow, all of which are vital for achieving your best.

I have personally used mental visualization techniques since 1982 to help me with my high school sports, college exams, weight training, public speaking, bodybuilding, musical performances, coaching youth sports, business deals, and more.

The power of positive thinking and visualization is simply amazing. You don't need to be an athlete or someone famous; it works for everyone. Give it a try.

"If you can imagine it, you can achieve it.
If you can dream it, you can become it."
~ William Arthur Ward,
20th century American writer

A Don Story: Visualization

With a fancy gold pen in my left hand, I was ready to sign the paperwork. My bank had just approved a large loan. Sitting in the title company's office, across from the seller and the realtor was surreal. It had been a long and tedious journey, but I was about to buy a building for my gym. Searching all over town for the previous four years had been quite a challenge. Either the space wasn't the right size or the cost was too steep, not to mention the need for ample parking.

At roughly the same square footage (about 5,500-square-feet) as my previous rental space, the new building was ideal. It had multiple windows, a high ceiling, lots of parking, and super visibility next to a frontage road that borders a very busy highway. None of these qualities existed at my old location. The old spot where I had been for 13-years (six years with Fitness Solutions 24/7 and seven with Flexers Gym) was the basement of a dilapidated old building. It had numerous plumbing and electrical problems, and the parking lot was like an ice-skating rink in the winter time.

The new space had been a restaurant for the past 25 years and would need a major overhaul. With the money now transferred from the bank into my account, we began the remodel in the spring of 2008. Stripping everything but the exterior, we hauled out old insulation, paneling, carpet, bricks, lighting fixtures, toilets, sinks, and more. Multiple large dumpsters were filled with the destruction. With tons of grease buildup on the concrete floor and metal ceiling area, where the kitchen hoods were located, muriatic acid was needed to get rid of the fatty slime that still smelled of old hamburgers, steaks, chicken, and French fries.

Once I got the approval for the loan, I knew the buildings dimensions by heart and could immediately start the process of the layout of equipment, locker rooms, office, lobby, etc. Having designed other fitness facilities in the past, I chose to do the design work myself. I actually love the process. With a bird's-eye view, drawing on graph paper, I sketched dozens of different options that I had visualized over years of planning. By visualizing the gym finished with all the touches that matter to me - great equipment, the right traffic flow, brightly painted walls, fresh flowers in the restrooms, potted plants - I could keep working at a steady pace with less stress.

For the entire four years that I searched for a building, I used visualization as a means to make my dream come true. Day and night I would picture different images and layouts of what I needed, wanted, and could afford. It certainly wasn't easy, but nothing worth having usually is.

Taking roughly three months to complete the demo, we were ready for the big move. Unlike the old white-walled, dungy, and dark basement of the old gym, this was a bright, colorful, and more welcoming facility. My dream came true.

"In order to make visualization a reality in the world form, you must be willing to do whatever it takes to make it happen."
~ Wayne Dyer, American philosopher

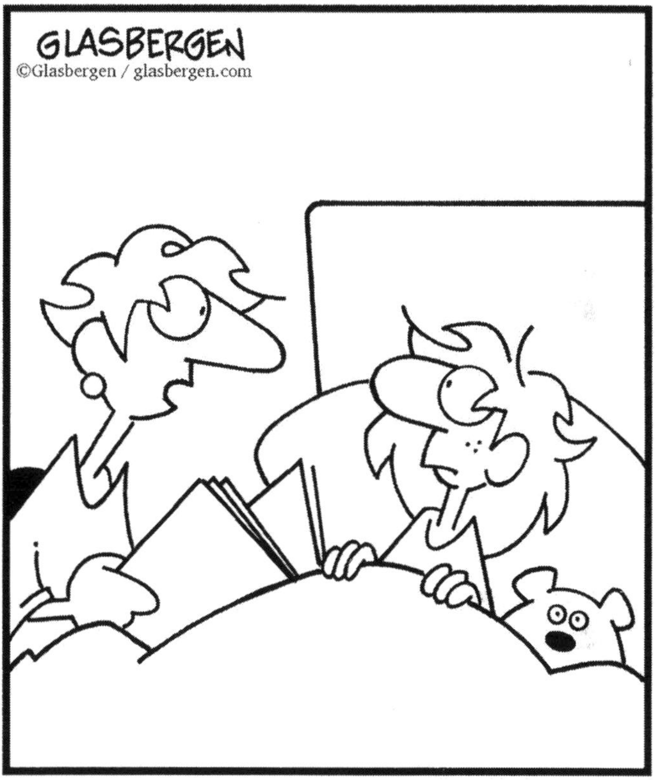

"It's different when you get older. When you're my age, visions of sugarplums dance on your thighs."

There are no proven ways for getting motivated to exercise.

Myth.

With so many challenges affecting our lives, whether at work or at home, it can be difficult getting motivated to exercise. While music and inspirational quotes are helpful tools in getting motivated, there are other scientifically proven methods to help you get fired up, says Deborah Feltz, PhD, a distinguished professor of kinesiology at Michigan State University and author of numerous fitness studies.

Make your workout a habit with these proven methods:

- **Write down your goals.** Those people who write down their goals and share them with a friend are 33% more likely to achieve that goal than someone who just talks about that same goal.
- **Don't use hard-and-fast rules.** "I must do an hour workout on Monday." This may be too difficult to maintain and thus makes it too easy to talk yourself out of the workout. Instead set yourself up for something small like a 15-30 minute workout at the gym or home.
- **Engage in some friendly competition.** This can be very helpful, even if you are not a competitive person. Find an individual or a group that is slightly better or faster than you. Nobody likes a quitter, even you.
- **Workout with a friend.** Accountability to someone besides yourself, who won't let you off

the hook, is very helpful. Having a workout buddy with similar goals can be exciting and fun.

- **Don't make exercise about how you look.** Not seeing changes in our physical appearance can be a downer. Instead focus on micro-goals that will help you celebrate small accomplishments, like doing a pull-up or a push-up. This should make you feel good and you should tell someone about your accomplishment.

A study published in *Health Psychology* found that people who used a "trigger" were more likely to actually follow through with their workout plans.

Here are some triggers that are popular:

- **Open up a big emotion.** Dedicate your workout to a cause greater than yourself, like a friend going through an illness, for an example.
- **Turn your complaining into appreciating.** Make it a challenge you want to do, rather than one you have to do.
- **Remind yourself how incredibly busy your life is.** It's now or never.
- **Try bribery.** Shopping for new clothes might do the trick.
- **Rethink your pajamas.** For an early morning workout, try sleeping in your workout clothes.

"People often say that motivation doesn't last.
Well, neither does bathing - that's why we recommend it daily."
~ Zig Ziglar, American author and motivational speaker

Keeping a journal for your exercise and nutrition records can double a person's weight loss.

Fact.

One third of American adults are obese! Two thirds of Americans are overweight or obese. Childhood obesity has more than doubled in the last 30 years. The financial toll of obesity on our healthcare system is greater than $190 billion per year. Read those statements again.

The following are findings from one of the largest and longest-running weight-loss maintenance trials, published in the *American Journal of Preventive Medicine* in August 2010. "The more food records people kept, the more weight they lost," said lead author Jack Hollis PhD, a researcher at Kaiser Permanente Center in Portland, Oregon. "Those who kept daily food records lost twice as much weight as those who kept no records." The six-month average weight loss was 13-pounds for nearly 1,700 participants. Two thirds (69%) lost at least nine pounds.

"If we all lost just nine pounds, our nation would be seeing a vast decrease in hypertension, diabetes, cholesterol, heart disease, and stroke," said study co-author, Victor Stevens PhD, a Kaiser Permanente researcher. In an earlier study, Stevens found that for every five pounds of weight loss, there was a 20% decrease in blood pressure.

The world's top athletes keep records of their progress in fitness and nutrition and these records become a source of inspiration for future accomplishments. There is no fooling yourself. Journaling your food helps develop positive lifestyle habits. You learn how to become aware of your physical and mental progress by monitoring your achievements.

Since 2002, Kaiser Permanente Care Management Institute on Weight Management has recommended maintaining an exercise and nutrition journal as an effective strategy for losing weight. The Weight Management Institute unites clinicians, researchers, insurers, and policymakers to identify practical, non-surgical approaches for the prevention and treatment of overweight and obese people.

Every day I hear clients say they can't lose weight. This study shows most people can lose weight if they have the right tools and support. "Food journaling in conjunction with a weight management program or class is the ideal combination of tools and support," says Keith Bachman, M.D., Weight Management Initiative member.

The study coordinated by the Portland, Oregon, Kaiser Permanente Center for Health and Research was also conducted at Duke University Medical Center, Pennington Biomedical Research Center, and Johns Hopkins University.

A fitness/nutrition journal can help you track:

- Changes in your mood
- Amount and quality of sleep you get
- Type and amounts of food you consume
- Type and amounts of exercise you perform
- Performance slumps in your exercise routine

I have personally used a fitness/nutrition journal since 2010. It has helped me manage my time better and attain the performance goals I have set for myself.

"What gets measured - gets done."
~ Lord Kelvin, Scots-Irish mathematical physicist and engineer

The best exercises for developing the calf muscles don't involve typical weight training exercises.

Fact.

Unless you are genetically gifted with muscular calves, you would probably agree that they are the most difficult muscles in the body to develop.

I am one of the many who have small calves, and while I have tried numerous strategies (high reps, low reps, stretching in between sets, etc.) for development, I have seen minimal change over the last thirty years of lifting. Is it possible that I, along with countless others have been going about it all wrong?

Since the calves get constant, low level stimulation all day from walking, they seldom respond to most activity. While many people use seated, standing, and inverted calf machines to develop these stubborn muscles, much of that time is being wasted by not using the most beneficial, yet uncommon, methods for developing these muscles of the lower legs.

If you look for the best calf development around, you will find that sprinters, soccer players, and volleyball players tend to have the best calf development. Interestingly, most of these athletes seldom use specific calf exercises as part of their weight training protocol.

Analyzing the muscle actions that these sports demand, the common component is deceleration. Whether changing directions on the field, landing on the floor, or slowing down from a top speed, all of these actions involve deceleration. This training involves what is known as the strength-shortening cycle.

According to Chad Waterbury, a neurophysiologist and coach for elite-level athletes, bodybuilders, and celebrities, paring calf exercises that train the strength-shortening and overload the eccentric (lengthening) phase of the muscle contraction is key. When partnered with a relatively high frequency of training each week (3-4 times), the results produce the greatest development for calf muscles.

Dr. Mel Siff says, "Concentrated sprinting and jumping exercises are more effective than a few sets of moderately heavy exercises on calf machines on providing training for stubborn calves. One should not forget that genetics have a major say in whether or not you can increase calf size dramatically."

Mark Kovac, a world-renowned performance physiologist says, "Doing some isolated work can be productive, but make sure it's a higher velocity isolated movement." Like Waterbury, Kovav recommends single-leg hops or taps instead of a calf raise machine. These movements allow you to isolate the calves in an explosive movement.

The following exercises can be done with bodyweight only, as I prefer, or holding a dumbbell on the same side. Staying on the ball of the foot is key as this will produce the greatest amount of load on the calf muscles. Jump as high as possible, minimizing landing time, while keeping knee flexion to a minimum.

Perform each of these non-traditional calf exercises with your knees straight, but not locked out.

Single-Leg Air Hops (my favorite)

- Stand on one leg with opposing leg bent
- Hop on one leg, spending as little time on the ground as possible
- Switch legs and repeat for the specified number of reps
- **Sets/Reps:** 2-5/10-30 each leg

Single-Leg Explosive Calf Raises

- Stand with one foot on a stair and your heel hanging off the step
- Keeping your knee straight, slowly lower your heel
- Forcefully extend your ankle as far as your range of motion allows
- Switch legs and repeat for the specified number of reps
- **Sets/Reps:** 2-5/10-30 each leg

Single-Leg Mini-Hurdle Hops

- Set up 6-8 hurdles in a straight line, about 2 feet apart
- Hop over the hurdles on one leg, spending as little time on the ground as possible
- Switch legs and repeat for the specified number of reps
- **Sets/Reps:** 2-5/5-10 each leg

Single-Leg Box Hops

- Stand on one leg with a 4-to-6 inch box in front of you
- Hop up to the box, extending your ankles to generate momentum
- Hop down and immediately repeat
- Switch legs and repeat for the specified number of reps
- **Sets/Reps:** 2-5/5-10 each leg

In addition to developing more muscular calves, these exercises also help with athletic performance.

"There are only two days in a year that nothing can be done. One is called yesterday and the other is called tomorrow."
~ The Dalai Lama

Jumping rope is far more effective than jogging for improving cardiovascular efficiency.

Fact.

A six-week study at Arizona State University, led by John A. Baker, showed that just 10-minutes of jumping rope was just as effective as jogging for 30-minutes for improving one's cardiovascular efficiency.

Jumping rope builds bone, balance, and muscles that most exercises can't match. Jumping rope burns over 1,000 calories per hour; rowing = 800, running = 600; walking = 400. Jumping rope incorporates muscles that move and those that hold the body stable. Jumping rope is a simple form of exercise that can be done almost anywhere.

It has been overshadowed for decades by fancy machines like treadmills, bikes, elliptical machines, and even running, but the fact remains that it has, and always will be, a superior form of exercise.

It's no wonder that boxers use it regularly. It is not easy, of course, unless you jumped rope growing up. Jumping rope requires skill, strength, focus, and patience. But once you master it, it can make you feel like a kid again.

Reasons to jump rope:

- Eliminate toxins by stimulating the lymphatic system (trash can of the body)
- Minimal equipment with easy transportation
- Tons of tricks to keep it interesting

- Simple, fast and convenient
- Warms you up quickly
- Full-body workout
- Do it anywhere
- Inexpensive
- Fun

According to Gray Cook, internationally known strength and conditioning specialist, Olympic weightlifting coach, and orthopedic and physical therapist, the collateral benefits of jumping rope complement the musculoskeletal system by improving posture and simulating the speed and reactions of any chosen sport.

With all the choices of equipment on the market today, many dismiss jumping rope as too simple and only minimally effective. Most chose plyometrics, as well as speed and agility work, thinking jumping rope is a waste of time. People who have never learned to jump rope or have a difficult time with technique may be embarrassed with their poor form, but this is precisely what makes jumping rope so effective. Rope jumping is hardly possible with poor form. By making constant small mistakes, like catching your foot, the rope becomes the coach.

The three basic movement patterns (foot positions) that are used in weight training, as well as most field and court sports, can be used in rope jumping:

- Squat stance: both feet placed side by side or slightly apart
- Lunge stance: one foot in front of the other, narrowing the base of support

- Hurdle step stance: single-leg stance in a stride position; one leg held out front (90 degrees) at the hip and knee

"Regardless of the skill level in any field or court sport, I recommend jumping rope as an excellent training tool that is both efficient and effective for reinforcing good movement patterns. Jumping rope will also help to develop great speed and agility and a power foundation for sports performance," says Cook.

Most of the impact of jumping rope is taken by your leg muscles. The erect posture and long spine needed for jumping rope, forces the core muscles to hold the midsection tight, forming the same kind of internal pressure as a weight belt.

Jumping rope forces you to use the ball of your foot versus the heel, which is how everyone should run, jump, and land to help prevent knee problems. Most knee injuries are non-contact. Jumping rope teaches the athlete to stay on the toes and be ready for action.

Cook recommends using 15, 20, or 30 second intervals as fast as you can, followed by twice the length of rest. Try to do this for at least four rounds.

Keep practicing. You'll get there. I used to hate jumping rope for the very reasons mentioned above. After a couple months of practicing a time or two per week, it became (and still is) one of my favorite methods of exercise.

"I don't have time" is the adult version of
"my dog ate my homework."
~ Unknown

Rebounding (jumping on a mini-trampoline) is as beneficial as jogging.

Fact.

This non-impact form of aerobic exercise produces greater biomechanical results and is less demanding than running. Much like its cousin, the jump rope, a mini-trampoline is 68% more efficient than jogging for the heart. A 1980 landmark study by NASA's Biomechanical Research Division published in the *Journal of Applied Physiology* shows this to be true. The American Council on exercise also states that jumping on a trampoline burns the same amount of calories as jogging.

This fun alternative form of exercise helps improve balance as well as increase spatial awareness, reducing the risk of falls later in life.

Rebounding bathes every cell in the body. By stimulating the lymphatic system, waste products are carried away. Without movement, these cells are left stewing in waste and starving for nutrients. Jumping on a mini-trampoline increases the lymphatic flow by 15-30 times. This effect can be beneficial for arthritis, cancer, and other degenerative diseases.

Rebounding stimulates all of the body's internal organs and moves cerebrospinal fluid. In turn, all cells become stronger, due to the increase in g-force. This cellular exercise makes immune cells up to five times more active, killing viruses, bacteria, and even cancer.

According to Albert Carter, the world's foremost authority on rebound exercise and professional trampolinist, "You can get all the aerobic exercise you need on a rebounder, and get all the lymphatic circulation you need on a rebounder, without the shock and trauma of hitting a hard surface."

Rebounding:

- Improves bone mass
- Helps improve balance
- Supports the thyroid and adrenal glands
- Enhances the benefits of other workouts
- Improves muscle tone throughout the body
- Boosts lymphatic drainage and immune system
- Helps circulate oxygen throughout the body to increase energy

I have used rebounding as part of my own warm-up for the past decade. As much as I prefer jumping rope, my knees sometimes can't handle the impact of rope jumping. If you feel like mixing things up, doing high and low jumps with alternative lateral arm swings on a mini-trampoline provides a fabulous variation to running, jumping rope, or box jumping.

"Don't accept average. It's just as far from the bottom as it is from the top."
~ Unknown

Whole Body Vibration is a useless method of exercise.

Myth.

Also known as Accelerated Vibration Training, Whole Body Vibration has become one of the fastest growing elements in fitness. Used in senior fitness centers, professional sports, and gyms, Whole Body Vibration has proven to be effective at every level of fitness. Vibration training exercises have actually been around since the times of the ancient Greeks, who used vibration instability training for developing better strength and balance for soldiers.

Working as the chief medical officer at the Battle Creek Sanitarium around 1900, John Harvey Kellogg, the co-creator of Kellogg's Cereal Company, used various forms of vibration training chairs to help reduce symptoms of back pain, headaches, and constipation, in addition to providing exercise. Kellogg also believed that the vibrational chairs provided the body with increased oxygenation.

Russian scientists worked with and fine-tuned vibration technology for years and then used it to rehabilitate their cosmonauts after they returned from space. This odd form of exercise, which involves standing or sitting on a vibrating platform, helped to repair muscles from atrophy and decreased bone density, due to weightlessness found in outer space. Vibration training enabled the Russians to stay in space 250 or more days, which was longer than their American counterparts. Vibration training helped the subjects reverse the effects of low gravity and improve muscle strength. Whole Body Vibration was also used to prevent injury in Russian Olympic athletes. If an athlete was injured, Whole Body Vibration was used to rehabilitate that injury. Eastern bloc countries continued using this method of vibration training into the 1970s in preparation for Olympic competition.

Since 2000, the popularity of Whole Body Vibration has grown tremendously in fitness facilities, private homes, therapy centers, and professional sporting facilities around the globe. The machine is a platform that is normally positioned six to eight inches off the floor and typically has handles for ease of use and safety. Various times and intensities may be programmed into the device.

Whole Body Vibration is one of the best ways to improve your lymphatic system. The lymphatic or "immune system" circulates lymphatic fluid through a system of tubes much like your arteries and veins. These tubes include a series of one-way valves. The vibration pumps the lymphatic fluid, allowing it to circulate properly.

Whole Body Vibration is recommended for cancer patients, anyone going through chemotherapy, or anyone with lymphedema. Whole Body Vibration helps the lymphatic system eliminate poisons and toxins from your body and strengthens each and every cell in your body, including cells in the liver, kidneys, bladder, heart, and lungs.

Externally, your skin will smooth and tighten, giving you a natural facelift. At the peak of every bounce, each cell in your body is suspended for a split second in a state of weightlessness. At the bottom of every bounce, each cell is receiving as much as two-to-four times normal gravitational force. Your whole body gets 1,200-3,600 impulses, stresses, or muscle contractions per minute with Whole Body Vibration. Every time you land on a rebounder (vibration machine, mini-tramp, or jumping rope) your body or cells want to collapse upon impact, but instead your cells must resist. This resistance is what builds cellular strength.

Jim Keller, a former Denver Broncos trainer and the founder of Next Level Sports Performance, swears by it. "Man-to-man, eye-to-eye, this is the best thing I've seen." The Green Bay Packers, Chicago Bulls, Manchester United, Sting, and Hilary Swank all use Whole Body Vibration regularly. Whole Body Vibration is especially good for obese people as it is a very low impact exercise.

Whole Body Vibration has been shown in the laboratory to provide the following benefits:

- Decreased cortisol
- Decreased body fat
- Decreased cellulite
- Decreased lower back pain
- Increased lymphatic drainage
- Increased growth hormone
- Increased muscle strength
- Increased bone mass
- Increased circulation
- Increased flexibility

"A year from now you'll wish you had started today."
~ Unknown

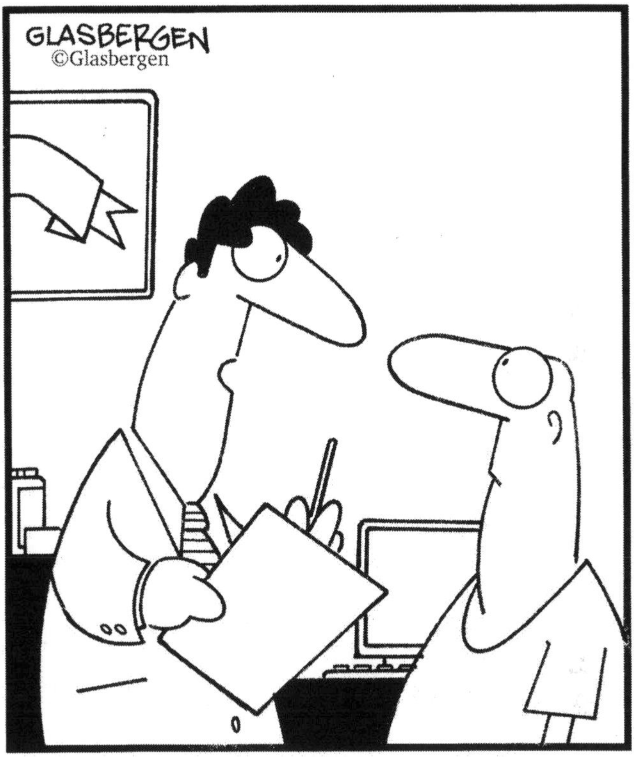

"The good news is, you have the heart of a teenager. The bad news is, most teenagers these days have the heart of an old man."

Jack LaLanne (1914-2011) was the greatest pioneer in the world of fitness.

Fact.

Known as the "Godfather of Fitness," Jack LaLanne was an American fitness, nutrition, and exercise guru, as well as a motivational speaker. He literally inspired millions to live a healthful life. He has most certainly inspired me.

However, he didn't start out healthy. As a teenager, he dropped out of school for a year because he was so ill. Thin, weak, and sickly, he even wore a back brace. "I also had blinding headaches every day," LaLanne recalled. "I wanted to escape my body because I could hardly stand the pain. My life appeared hopeless." LaLanne was a sugar and junk food addict with anger and behavioral problems.

At 15 years old, after hearing a motivational, nutritional talk by Paul Bragg, a pioneer nutritionist, LaLanne stopped his sugar addiction and turned his life around. He started eating healthfully and lifting weights.

LaLanne believed the country's overall health depended on the health of the population. He believed nutrition and physical fitness were "the salvation of America." LaLanne published numerous books on fitness and hosted the Jack LaLanne show from 1953 to 1985, the longest-running television exercise show of all time. In 1936, at the age of 21, he opened one of the nation's first gyms in Oakland, California. This became the prototype for dozens of similar gyms bearing his name.

"People thought I was a charlatan and the nut," LaLanne said. Doctors were against him and said things like, "Weights will give people heart attacks." He encouraged women to join health clubs. LaLanne invented numerous exercise machines that are still used today, including the cable pulley, the Smith Machine, and the leg extension machine.

He coached elderly and disabled to enhance their strength. LaLanne was a bodybuilder and a strong man. At the age of 54, and standing only 5'6", he beat Arnold Schwarzenegger, 6'3 and 21 at the time, in an informal bodybuilding contest. He was inducted into the California Hall of Fame and the Hollywood Walk of Fame.

Here are just a few of Jacks amazing feats:

- Could do one-armed fingertip pushups while in a completely stretched out position.
- 1955 (age 40), swam from Alcatraz to Fisherman's Wharf in San Francisco while handcuffed.
- 1956 (age 41), set a world record of 1,033 push-ups in 23-minutes on "You Asked for It" TV program.
- 1960 (age 45), did 1,000 jumping jacks and 1,000 chin-ups in one-hour 22-minutes to promote the Jack LaLanne show going nationwide. He said this was the most difficult stunt he had done; difficult only because the skin on his hands started ripping off from the chin-ups!

- 1965 (age 60), swam from Alcatraz to Fisherman's Wharf in San Francisco for a second time. This time he not only wore handcuffs, but also towed a 1,000 pound boat.

Even at 94, Jack was still exercising daily. It was his consistency that made LaLanne superhuman. His daily habits led to his long-term success.

"Physical fitness takes commitment to exercise just as it requires good nutrition. But it doesn't have to be painful. Just the opposite: Vigorous exercise actually is stimulating. It boosts your energy levels, invigorates your mind, and just feels good afterward. The hardest part, of course, is getting started."

~ Jack LaLanne

No trainer in history has brought more to bodybuilding than Vince Gironda (1917-1997).

Fact.

Many of you may know the name Joe Weider. He was touted as the "Trainer of Champions." However, a much lesser known figure had one of the most successful following of bodybuilding champions. His name is Vince Gironda, and he opened the third gym in America, in Hollywood, after Jack LaLanne in San Francisco and Sig Klein in New York City.

Vince was known as the "Iron Guru" and "Trainer to the Stars," because he got actors in shape fast for their roles. He trained numerous famous bodybuilders including Arnold Schwarzenegger, Lou Ferrigno, Frank Zane, and Larry Scott. He was against the use of steroids, but unfortunately all of his professional bodybuilding clients used them. He also trained dozens of movie stars including Clint Eastwood, Cher, Robert Blake, Denzel Washington, Sean Penn, Eric Estrada, and James Garner. Many people haven't heard of him because he didn't market himself like Weider did. Vince was very honest and direct, which some big-ego bodybuilders didn't like. He once told the young, pompous, and husky Arnold Schwarzenegger that he was fat!

Vince realized that certain exercises were better than others for proper muscular development. For example, the bench press is actually a poor chest exercise. It over stimulates the anterior deltoid and tricep muscle. Some gym goers train on the bench press to impress others. "Hey dude, how much do you bench?" The dumbbell press (flat and incline), dips, and cable machine are all superior to the bench press for chest development.

Analyzing the anatomy and exact function of a muscle and then finding the right variation to target that muscle was arguably Vince's greatest contribution.

Vince was the first trainer to talk about intensity to build muscle and lose fat. This method involves doing more work in less time. Even though not great for strength, this method results in greater mass. Vince recommended rest time between sets to be short, at only 15-seconds. It is best to start with longer rest periods if you are used to doing one-to-three minute rests. Gradually decrease your rest time to increase intensity. In order to accomplish this you must use less weight. Eventually, that weight will go back up, once you're accustomed to the new method.

Vince recommended this method as early as the 1950s and 1960s. In 1925, German scientists discovered that to enlarge muscles you must increase intensity within a specific time. This method later became known as German Volume Training (GVT). Vince never claimed to be the sole inventor, but he likely discovered this principle himself through trial and error. Unlike GVT's 10-sets of 10-reps method with one minute of rest between sets, which is a very tough workout for bodybuilding, Vince's method used eight-sets of eight-reps followed by only 30 seconds of rest, which is even more strenuous.

In the 35 plus years that I have been personally training, I have only met a few men and women with the mental and physical toughness to do these incredibly intense workouts.

They are some of my personal favorites for natural bodybuilding, but not part of my regular programs for the general public. Vince also popularized low-carb eating, known as the "meat and eggs diet" long before Atkins and others were even known.

"If you don't like what you see in the mirror, what difference does it make what the scale says?"
~ Vince Gironda

A Don Story: Main Street Gym

Peering into what seemed to be a retail store, I assumed I had entered the wrong door. Walking back outside to the sidewalk, I looked around. To the north was Parson's Drug Store and to the south was Wallace Furniture. I glanced up again at the sign overhead: "Main Street Gym." A curved olympic barbell was the logo and "Gym is Tonic" was the tagline.

As I returned back into the space, I noticed Kachina dolls and other odd items on the shelves. Next to them were stacks of Indian rugs, racks of swimsuits, T-shirts, pants, and other clothing. What kind of a gym was this? Had the gym moved to another location? I saw no bodies sweating, nor did I hear any heavy breathing or weights. The faint sound of classic rock music was the only audio. There were no weights or other fitness items to be seen from my vantage point. Continuing down the old wooden floor were free weights, weight machines, a couple pieces of cardio equipment, and some boxing equipment. With a rather tall ceiling of roughly 20-feet, there was even a partial basketball court in the corner. This was by far the strangest gym I had ever seen or heard of, albeit my experiences were limited to only a handful.

As I continued my solo tour, I could see the facility had all the basic equipment that I was accustomed to. With a reasonable monthly rate and no contracts, I figured I could afford the price. Like the Del Norte High School weight room and the Fort Lewis College gym, the Main Street Gym became my lifting sanctuary.

In 1992, to my elation, I took over as their head trainer, replacing a woman who had been a popular trainer there for the previous few years. Even though I wasn't making much money, I knew I had found my calling. Educating, motivating and inspiring people through fitness and nutrition was my new passion, born and nurtured years ago in Del Norte High School.

I learned quickly that the owner of the Main Street Gym packed the entrance to his gym with Indian rugs and dolls, swimwear, T-shirts, sweatpants, supplements, and more to bring in more dollars. Selling gym memberships alone might not pay all the bills. So while training clients, I also needed to manage the front desk. Over the course of a shift, I would make multiple trips to and from the front sales counter to check members in and sell retail sales items. I learned early on what it took a make a dollar in the gym business, a lesson that served me well when I opened Fit 24/7.

"Muscles are the badges that one can wear regardless of their gender, race, religion, political affiliation, or social status."
~ Unknown

The psoas may be the most important muscle in the body.

Fact.

A Greek word meaning "the loin region," the mighty psoas muscle is responsible for many key functions. This deepest muscle in your core is attached above at the lumbar spine and below on the pelvis. This long, spindle-like muscle joins the upper and lower body together. Without this muscle, you wouldn't be able to get out of bed in the morning.

Whether you bike, run, ski, hike, or just sit on your couch, your psoas muscles are involved. The psoas forms our hip flexors and is instrumental in controlling flexion of the hip joint. This deep-seated muscle supports our core and is important for proper postural function. If the psoas is weak, one can experience back pain and mechanical problems. Known as the "muscle of the soul," many believe it is also important for emotional, as well as spiritual health.

Olympic weightlifters, runners, triathletes, and gymnasts all rely heavily on the psoas for support. Linked to the spinal cord and brain stem, this key messenger for the central nervous system, connects to the diaphragm through fascia (connective tissue), which affects both breathing and our fear reflex.

Liz Koch, a psoas expert and author of *The Psoas Book,* states that emotional trauma or lack of emotional support can lead to a chronic contracted psoas, which transfers to a lack of core awareness.

A healthy psoas is vital for:

- Healthy posture
- Healthy lower back
- Optimal sports performance
- A more pain-free pregnancy

A tight psoas is caused by:

- A weak core
- Chronic sitting
- Doing lots of sit-ups
- Poor neuromuscular control
- Prolonged bicycling or running

A dysfunctional psoas (short and tight) may lead to a host of kinetic chain problems:

- Sway back
- Low back pain
- Hip impingement
- Shallow breathing
- Hamstring strains
- Sacroiliac (SI) joint pain
- Knee pain (patellar tendinitis)
- Anterior pelvic tilt (Piriformis Syndrome)

Consult a physical therapist or other specialist with experience on releasing the psoas if you are experiencing any of these symptoms. Practicing self massage (myofascial release) with a foam roller or a Theracane is strongly recommended to maintain psoas health. These are both part of my weekly protocol for keeping my psoas stretched and healthy. Stretching the surrounding hip muscles (hip flexor stretch, kneeling lunge stretch), as well as strengthening the glutes (ball or floor bridge, split squats, etc.) and core (planks, dying bug, leg lifts, etc.) are all vitally important for psoas integrity. Yoga and Pilates may be an avenue of help for you, as well.

Although surgery is often prescribed for back pain, and still may be necessary, researchers are finding that focusing on improving the health of the psoas muscle can dramatically reduce low back pain.

I can attest to a tight psoas being partially, if not totally responsible for my low back problems, hamstring pulls, and knee pain over the past 35 years.

"Fitness is not about being better than someone else,
it's about being better than you used to be."
~ Unknown

Scientists have found a new organ called fascia; it could be the largest in your body.

Fact.

How can it be possible that medical professionals have missed this for all these years? Fascia (interstitium) is the thin, fibrous, fluid-filled connective tissue surrounding every muscle and organ in your body from head to toe. This tissue is like a honeycomb from the inside of the body out to the skin.

"Techniques in processing tissue from surgery and biopsies failed to identify this space because it was artificially collapsed during the fixation process, or when tissue is prepared to view under a microscope," the journal *Scientific Reports* stated.

I like to use the comparison of a grapefruit. Think of the peel as the skin. Once the peel is removed and you section the grapefruit (or other citrus), look at the membrane that surrounds the juice within; this membrane is similar to fascia. Without this membrane, the grapefruit would have no structural integrity and would fall apart, just as our body would without fascia. The juice represents the muscles that are full of water.

Dr. Neil Theise, professor of pathology at NYU Langone Health in New York and co-senior author of the study, states, "Initially, we were just thinking it's an interesting tissue, but when you actually delve into how people define organs, it sort of runs around one or two ideas: that it has a unitary structure, or it's a tissue with a unitary function."

Theise goes on to say, "I think it's bigger than the skin," which makes up roughly 16% of our body and was considered the largest organ until recently. His estimate is that 20% of the body is fascia!

Dr. Michael Nathanson, Yale University School of Medicine Professor of Medicine and Cell Biology and Section Chief of Digestive Diseases and not involved in the study stated, "In my opinion, this has the potential to change our understanding of the human body because this 'pre-lymphatic region,' as the authors refer to it, may undergo changes in certain disease states such as certain types of cancer . . . So this now puts us in a position to figure out whether this is an effect or else perhaps part of the cause of such diseases."

This newfound network is a passageway for lymph, the vital fluid for the functioning of immune cells that generate inflammation. The cells that reside in this network change with age, and may contribute to the stiffening of limbs, wrinkling of skin, and numerous diseases.

"We are optimistic that with what we learned, we'll soon be able to study and target the interstitial space for diagnosis of disease and perhaps for novel personalized treatments," wrote co-lead author, Dr. Petros Constantinos Benias from the Feinstein Institute and Zucker School of Medicine at Hofstra/Northwell Health.

Why having healthy fascia is important:

- **Fascia is like a sponge.** If it dries out, facia becomes hard and brittle and can break with little force. If this fascial tissue is well hydrated, the results are greater mobility, integrity, and resilience. When water is absent, the muscles stick together. If they are dry, they are more inclined to erode, tear, or rupture. However, more water alone doesn't work. Like a kink in a hose, we need to work on the fascia and untangle the sticky sections. Bodyworkers who specialize in myofascial work (Rolfing and other deep-tissue, structural integrity methods) are recommended for acute problems. Having been Rolfed over a dozen times, I will tell you first-hand that it and other deep-tissue work can be extremely uncomfortable, and even painful, yet very beneficial. Foam rollers, myofascial balls, tennis balls, lacrosse balls, Thera Canes, golf balls, hand rollers, and more, are all helpful, as well. The problem is that most people don't want to make themselves uncomfortable. If someone else is doing the myofascial treatment on you, it seems to be more bearable.

- **Variable movement patterns help hydrate fascia**. Intense exercise drives the water out of the tissue. Rest is how the tissue rehydrates. When you take the pressure away from the tissue (rest), like a sponge, the fascia will soak up the water and be ready for more exercise. Exercise followed by rest, followed by exercise, followed by rest, is the cycle that maintains healthy fascia.
- **All of the fascial tissue, from head to toe, is connected**. A problem in one area of your body can affect other parts of the body. Many people use the example of a sweater to demonstrate the effect. Grabbing one end of the sweater will stretch the other end. A neck injury leads to a

shoulder injury, and then years later, that shoulder injury leads to a lower back injury. I know this all too well, because it happened to me with my neck and back. Years of collisions on the gridiron, coupled with years of non-variable patterns in my exercise routine and minimal stretching/bodywork was a recipe for injury and pain. I herniated a disc twenty-five years ago, which forced me to look at various techniques like deep-tissue massage, chiropractic, Rolfing, and more. To this day, if I am lazy about my foam rolling and stretching, neglecting these exercises for three-to-seven days, my back will go out. Additionally, shoveling dirt or snow on only one side of my body, can be problematic. Riding a road bicycle, with the neck and back rounded, may also cause problems. Sitting at a desk or in a car for long periods can also be an issue. The best way to prevent this dreaded domino effect is to keep the fascia healthy.

- **Healthy fascial tissue is optimal for athletes and couch potatoes alike.** Having healthy fascial tissue means less muscle power is needed for the same task, which in turn equals less fatigue. To run faster, lift heavier, jump higher, throw further, hike longer, and ski better, you must have healthy fascia. Like a built-in trampoline effect, it is best to incorporate more bouncy movements into your routines. Jumping rope, box jumps, kickboxing, and martial arts will all help maintain healthy fascia.

- **Healthy fascia is vital for proper alignment and function, keeping injuries from becoming chronic**. This newly identified organ, the largest in the human body, is said to have six-to-ten times the sensory nerve receptors that muscles have and about the same number as the retina of our eye. Keeping your fascia healthy can help you avoid surgery and/or joint replacement.

"The fascia forms the largest system in the body as it is the system that touches all the other systems."
~ James L. Oschman, PhD, biological sciences

Static stretching is an outdated methodology that should not be used.

Myth.

Static stretching means a stretch is held in a challenging but comfortable position for a period of time, usually 10-30 seconds. I recommend 30-60 seconds and even 90 seconds if a muscle is extremely tight. This most common form of stretching has gotten a bad rap.

Alwyn Cosgrove, a world renowned fitness expert says, "We over-react in the short term and under-react in the long term." Static stretching went from being the "best" way to stretch to "don't do at all." 1980s results showed that static stretching could decrease an athlete's power (albeit minimal), which led to people over-reacting and to the birth of dynamic warm-up. This had positive and negative effects.

Dynamic flexibility has been huge in the performance world of athletes of all types. But static stretching can have solid benefits when implemented properly, according to Eric Cressey, Strength and Conditioning Specialist. The reality is that static stretching is not good in and of itself, but when combined with dynamic flexibility or an "active warm-up," it becomes a superior technique. An active warm-up is the best way to prevent an injury. Doing dynamic movements before practice, games, and lifting weights has been proven to decrease hamstring and groin pulls.

Lack of flexibility can spell trouble for many athletes with problems like knee pain, low back pain, and shoulder pain. Many people believe that dynamic movement as a pre-workout and static stretching as a post workout is best. Not so. According to Michael Boyle, one of the world's most qualified strength and conditioning coaches, post workout stretching does not increase flexibility. Static stretches followed by a dynamic warm-up best prepares the muscles for a workout.

To further enhance the benefits of this protocol, it is advised to do foam rolling before stretching and dynamic movements to lengthen the tissue.

- **Foam Roll** (3-5 minutes) - to decrease the density of the muscle. Muscle responds to injury and overuse by increasing in density. This leads to a knot or trigger point. Foam rolling has many names: Massage, ART (Active Release Technique), MAT (Muscle Activation Technique), STM (Soft Tissue Mobilization), and more. All these methods are used to change the density of the muscle. Foam rolling is a "poor man's massage." It is a great way to get changes in the muscle tissue before stretching. Think of it as ironing the muscles.
- **Static Stretching** (3-5 minutes) - do after foam rolling and before dynamic movement. Most soft tissue experts recommend stretching a cold muscle without warming up. Simply roll and then stretch. A warm muscle elongates and then returns to normal length. A cold muscle undergoes deformation and increases in length. Stretching can be hard, boring, and time consuming, but is important.

- **Dynamic movement** (3-5 minutes) - do after foam rolling and static stretching. Jumping jacks, seal jacks, rowing machine, agility ladder, slide board, burpees, Jacob's Ladder, ball slams, and much more, are all examples of dynamic movement.

Now you are ready to workout with maximum effectiveness and the least likelihood of injury.

"If you stretch regularly, you will find that every movement you make becomes easier."
~ Bob Anderson, author and stretching expert

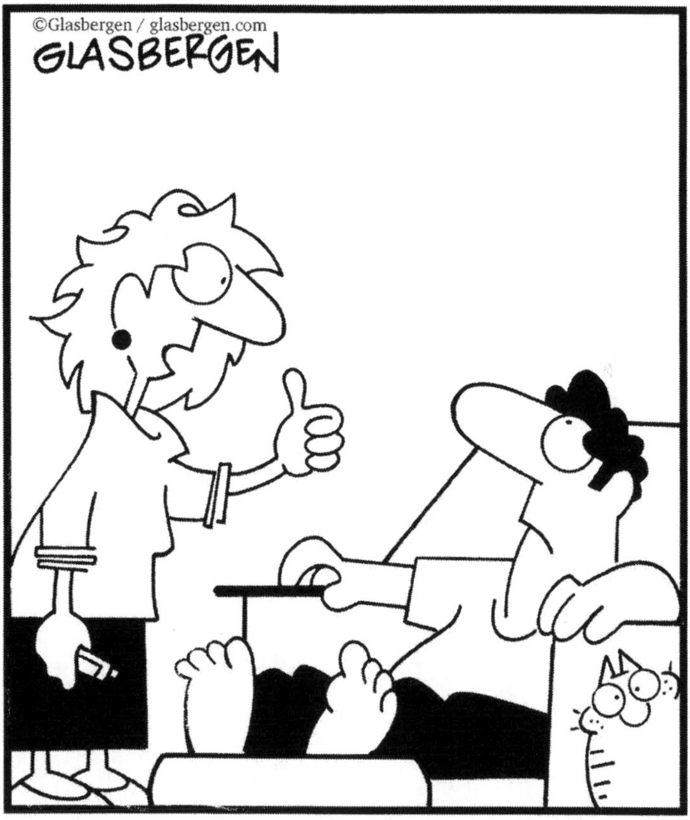

"You need to incorporate some stretching into your fitness routine, so I glued all of your snacks to the ceiling!"

Couples who train together tend to stay together.

Fact.

Across the globe, individuals are hitting the gym, running, bicycling and signing up for fitness challenges. You may want to consider training with your significant other. Exercise not only benefits your own well-being, but also that of your romantic partner. A number of studies are showing that couples who sweat together really do stay together.

"When a couple works out together, the actual exercise itself can physically and emotionally have a positive impact," says marriage and relationship psychotherapist Dr. Jane Greer. "Both partners come away with feelings of synchronicity, cooperative spirit, and shared passion. Then you throw in some spicy endorphins and it can be a real power trip for the relationship." The research shows surprising benefits from couples who work out together.

Enjoying shared physical activities together:

- **Increases happiness within your relationship** - Couples report feeling more satisfied with their relationship and more in love with their partner. Exercise induces symptoms of arousal with a racing pulse, sweaty hands, and shortness of breath.
- **Improves the efficiency of your workouts** - The presence of someone else affects your ability to do an activity. Your partner's presence may improve your speed subconsciously.

- **Helps you achieve your fitness goals** - It's easier to achieve your fitness goals when your partner cares about their own goals, as well as yours. Training together keeps one another accountable and motivated.
- **Increases your emotional bond** - Working out together can help coordinate your actions, whether lifting weights, rowing, biking, walking, hiking or running.
- **Improves your sex life** - Your heart rate, digestion, and libido all improve with exercise. Exercise can actually double your desire for physical intimacy.

Twenty percent of the members that have been at my facility for over 15 years are couples.

"Fitness is like marriage.
You can't cheat on it and expect it to work."
~ Unknown

13-minute weight training workouts are sufficient for developing muscular strength and endurance.

Fact.

In this hustle and bustle world, the number one reason people state for not joining a gym is "time." Trying to fit an hour workout into your busy schedule can seem like a daunting task. But now we know that effective weight training workouts can be done in as little as 13-minutes. The greater the intensity of the exercise you perform, the less time is needed to accomplish effective results. The excuse of lack of time just got weaker.

One set of weight training to failure is enough to build muscular strength and endurance, according to a new study conducted by researchers at Lehman College in the Bronx.

The study used 34 fit young men who did regular resistance training. Research tested for muscular strength, size, and endurance and then randomly assigned them to three supervised weight-training routines.

The basic program consisted of seven common exercises, including the machine leg press, lat pull-down, bench press, and others. One set of each of these exercises was completed to failure (muscular exhaustion) within eight to twelve repetitions. The number of sets for each group differed. One group did five sets of each exercise with roughly 90 seconds of rest between sets. Their complete session lasted about 70 minutes. A second group did three sets of each exercise and trained for about 40 minutes. The third group only did one set of each exercise and was done after only 13 minutes.

Each volunteer trained three times per week for a total of eight weeks and then was remeasured for results. After two months, all of the men were stronger. Surprisingly, the strength improvements were the same, regardless of how many - or few sets the men performed. The groups showed equal improvements in muscular endurance as well, measured by using a bench press exercise with low weight. The size of the men's muscles were in fact different. Those who had performed five sets per session showed the greatest increase in muscle mass.

My full-body workouts are tried and true, having been used for the last three decades with my male and female clients of all ages. And they aren't just for beginners. With increased intensity and short rest time, intermediates and advanced weight trainers also benefit from short, intense, full-body workouts.

You won't see any calf raises, bicep curls, leg extensions, tricep extensions, leg curls, or other isolation movements that only use one joint. These exercises only recruit a fraction of the muscles that the compound movements do.

My mini-workouts, as I call them, primarily incorporate big compound movements (like squats, deadlifts, swings, planks, rows, and chest press) that utilize two or more joints at a time (hips and knees or shoulders and elbows), recruiting the most muscle tissue and elevating the metabolism to its fullest.

Done in a circuit, several exercises can be completed in a fraction of the time that normal workouts take.

The benefits of doing these mini-workouts are:

- Saving time
- Staying motivated
- Increased strength
- Improving your memory
- Simplifying your workouts
- Increasing anabolic hormones
- Increasing cardiovascular efficiency

"A 15-minute workout is 1% of your day. No excuses!"
~ Unknown

Don's Home/Travel Workout

Eighty-five percent of Americans don't make the time to go to the gym. There are actually a significant number of exercises that can be done in the privacy of your own home, office, hotel room, or outside. These require little to no equipment, minimal space, and can be done two-to-three times a week for 15-30 minutes each time. It's about recruiting big muscle groups with minimal rest. This spells INTENSITY!

- **Body squats** - Arms out, butt back, chest forward, eyes forward. Don't round the back. Keep the heels on the floor. Keep knees in line with toes. Jump to increase intensity.
- **Band rows** - Sit on the floor with both legs extended. Wrap the band around the bottom of both feet. Keep spine straight, knees soft, engage your core, and squeeze shoulder blades together. Wrap the band around a solid bedpost or both door knobs of an open door (or other stable structure) as an alternative. Best to use a band with handles. Moderate to heavy bands are recommended.
- **Reverse lunges** - One foot steps backward, keeping front knee just above toes. Return forward and repeat with opposite leg. Hold on to counter or doorknobs of an open door for support, if needed. The majority of your weight should be on the front leg. The back leg is primarily for balance.

- **Push-ups** (on knees, if necessary) - Fingers straight ahead and next to chest at the bottom of the movement. Keep spine straight. Look at floor instead of up.
- **Supermans** - Lying face down, lift your arms and legs off the floor. Hold for a second or two and then relax. Look at the floor.
- **Planks** - On elbows or with arms extended, and on knees or toes. Alternate opposing legs and arms, if possible, to increase intensity. Keep spine straight. Look at the floor.

Do all of these exercises as a circuit (one after the other). Do AMRAP (as many reps as possible), slowly (2 to 4 seconds each direction), using good form. Control the motion. Don't let the motion control you! Do not hold your breath! With minimal rest, move onto the next exercise. This will double as a cardiovascular workout. Start with one-to-two sets and increase each week, if manageable (three-to-four sets max). Do this workout two-to-three times per week with a minimum of 48-hours (every other day) between each session. Throw a short hollow foam roller, a lacrosse ball or tennis ball (all for fascial massage), and a jump rope in your suitcase for added benefits.

"Your workouts are important meetings
you scheduled with yourself.
Bosses don't cancel."
~ Unknown

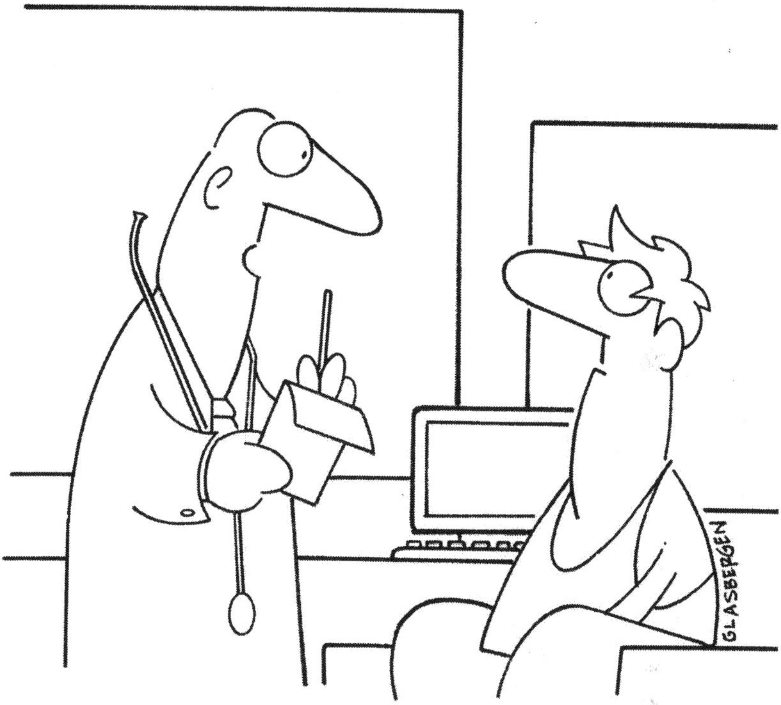

"I'm prescribing exercise. Think of it as a stress pill that takes 30 minutes to swallow."

Don's Fitness Tips and Reminders

- Prioritize weight training over cardiovascular exercise.
- Weight training in a paired or circuited fashion saves time and increases cardiovascular health in addition to building muscle and bone, strengthening muscle, and burning fat.
- Remember that free-weights are more functional (replicating real life movements) and recruit more muscle tissue than machines. Use dumbbells, barbells, kettlebells, TRX straps, and body-weight most of the time.
- Use primarily compound movements, that involve two or more joints, like squats, lunges, rows, chest presses, lat pulls, shoulder presses, and planks.
- Vary your exercises, sets, reps, speed, and rest time each workout to maximize gains in strength, hypertrophy (growth), and to minimize adaptation and boredom.
- Aim for three non-consecutive days (Monday, Wednesday and Friday, for example) per week for your training. More than this is not necessary, if you are on a well-balanced nutritional program.
- Plan your workouts ahead of time to make them more efficient and effective.

- A 10-15 minute warm-up that consists of foam rolling, stretching, and dynamic movement can do wonders for your performance in and out of the gym.
- Execute proper form before increasing the weight on any exercise.
- Listening to your favorite music can have a tremendous impact on motivation.
- Every exercise is not for everyone. Depending on your range of motion, length of limbs, skill-set, comfort level, injuries, and more, you should consult a fitness professional to establish the best choices for YOU!
- Use a weight that isn't too heavy or too light. Most women lift too light, while most men lift too heavy.
- If you think doing hundreds of pounds on the leg press machine is as effective as doing a fraction of that weight doing squats, lunges or deadlifts, we need to have a talk.
- Train smarter, not harder. Check your ego at the door.
- Progressive resistance plateaus at some point. Intensity is the name of the game.
- Women and men should do the same weight bearing exercises. Our muscular structure is almost identical. Ladies, you will get stronger and leaner.
- Cardio that utilizes upper and lower body together are best in my opinion: rower, airdyne bike, elliptical with arms, Jacob's ladder, jump rope, jumping jacks, burpees, etc.

- Use a fitness/nutrition journal to track your progress, to keep you accountable to yourself and/or your trainer, and to reach your goals.
- Harness the power of visualization to help you attain those goals.
- You can't out-exercise poor nutrition.
- Sleep seven-to-nine hours per night to maximize growth hormone (muscle builder) and minimize cortisol (fat storer).
- Get outside when possible. Walk, bike, hike, ski, garden, etc. We need the fresh air and sunshine to survive and thrive.
- Make fitness a priority. Health is your number one asset.

"You are only one workout away from a good mood."
~ Unknown

A Don Story: The Hassle of Moving

It was a gorgeous Saturday morning in early August of 2008. I was excited that we were about to move into the new gym facility in Bodo Park, just south of Durango. I was scheduled to meet the owner of the moving company I had hired at 8:30 am.

Introducing ourselves, he quickly handed me a clip board and asked for my signature. The start time on the paperwork showed 8:00. It was 8:30 and he wanted to be paid for drive time. At $100 per hour ($50 for the drive), this seemed unreasonable to me, and I quickly expressed my unease to him. We were already off to a bad start.

Waiting on his helpers to arrive and watching in disbelief as the owner repaired his broken dolly, I was concerned about the unsettling task ahead. Having never moved a big gym before, this guy had no idea what he was in store for.

After 30-minutes of watching him try to fix his dolly and working alongside one of his less-than-competent employees who finally arrived, I knew I had to make a change.

I called the local moving truck rental facility to inquire about a large moving truck with 10-foot ceilings. They had a 26-footer, but only with an eight-foot ceiling. This would have to do. Beggars can't be choosers, as they say. No other options presented themselves. Picking up the truck and driving back to the gym, I let the moving company's owner know that we no longer required his services. He didn't seem to care and left without any difficulty.

As the saying goes, friends are worth their weight in gold. If you ever ask someone to help you move and they really do help, you've got a true friend. This fine day, I had a half-dozen friends, and we needed every single one to accomplish this enormous job.

I had moved a gym twice before, but this was different. The amount of equipment was about double that of years past. With refrigerator dollies, piano dollies, hand trucks, drills, wrenches, screwdrivers, pry bars and more, we began. Some of it was as easy as just picking up various dumbbells, barbells, and plates. Other pieces were more complicated, as they had to be disassembled and put on a dolly.

The trickiest of all were the large weight machines: assisted chin/dip; crossover cable; leg extension; leg curl; etc. that were roughly 8-feet tall and had to be moved as a unit without disassembling. Some of these machines weighed as much as 800 pounds. I preferred a truck with a 10-foot high ceiling to enable the machines to be placed upright. Laying them on their backs was far more work and took up much more floor space.

These pieces were on ½ inch rubber flooring and when trying to roll a 400-800 pound item across such flooring, the results were waves of rubber blocking the small dolly wheels from rolling. After trying numerous methods, we discovered that strips of cardboard placed under the wheels did the trick most of the time. Sometimes, all of us would grab a side and hoist and carry the monstrosity to its temporary destination inside the big truck. Carrying 100-150 pounds each for long distances is incredibly taxing on the body.

As brutal as it was to load the moving truck at the old location, the real trial was unloading it at the new one. The old location had a loading dock that made the transfer from building to truck only somewhat arduous, because of the 6-inch height variation. The new location had no such dock and the sidewalk outside the door was about 4-feet lower than the bed of the truck. We would need to use the trucks long and narrow aluminum ramp to unload.

With one person at the far end of the strapped dolly, and one at the other, we proceeded to try what none of us had done before. With the ramp less than 3-feet wide, we couldn't fit more than one person at each end of the big machines. The others would stay below and try to help from each side of the ramp in case we lost control. When an item that weighs several hundred pounds is influenced by momentum going down a ramp that drops several feet in a short amount of time, the results can be dangerous and disastrous.

Working from early in the morning to late into the night, we spent three long days hauling multiple loads to and from. From the marathon of pushing, pulling and dragging, we were all physically and mentally exhausted. Muscles and heads ached; hands and fingers blistered and bled; but fortunately, nobody was injured. I'm convinced that had we not all been in such good shape from years of lifting weights, we may have suffered numerous injuries. The new gym was now ready for its unveiling.

"For the price of a one-year gym membership,
you can replace your entire wardrobe with larger clothes."
~ Unknown

Section Two

Don's Clients Photos and Testimonials

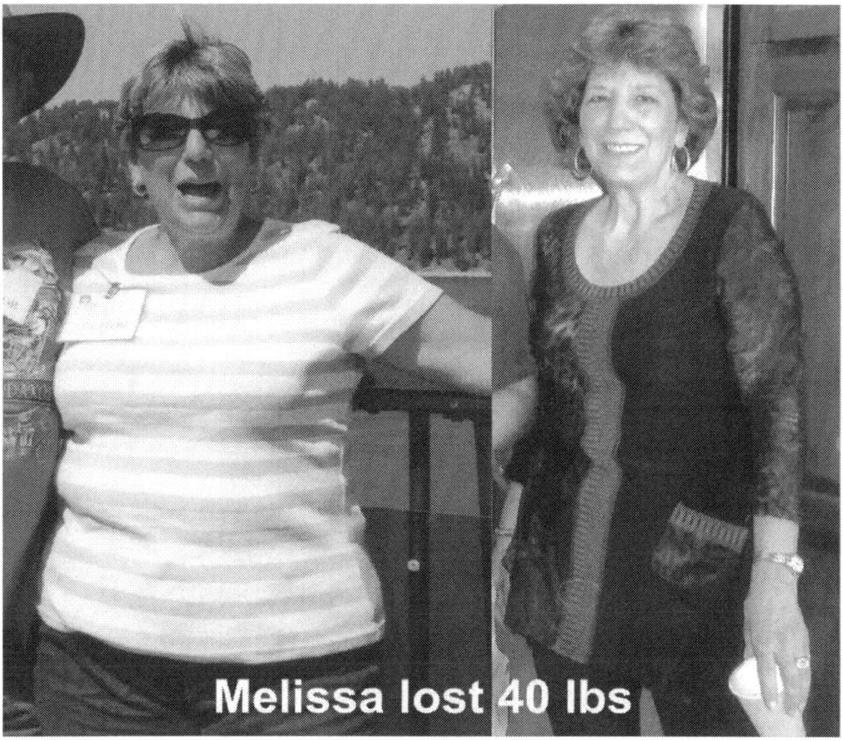

"Throughout my life, my weight has fluctuated 30-40 pounds. Don's revolutionary exercise and eating program enlightened me to a totally different way of thinking about both. I lost 40-pounds, gained muscle tone and downsized from a size 14 to a size 10. No kidding! I still eat ice cream, lattes, and red wine, just not every day." **~ Melissa Klumph, client and Fit 24/7 gym member**

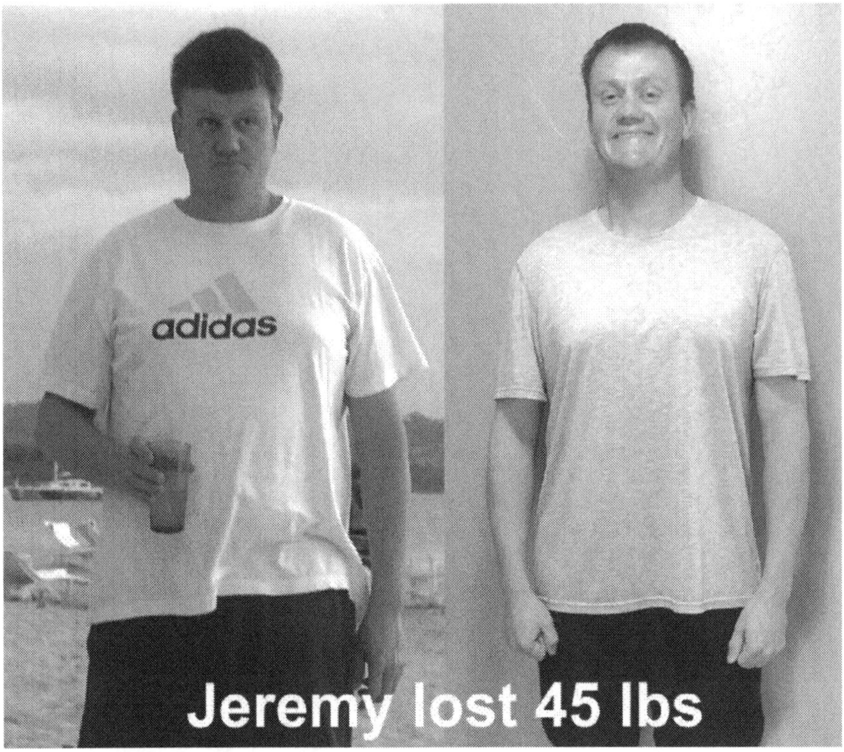

"I first came to Fit 24/7 at 230 lbs. Two years later, I now weigh 185 lbs. It's pretty crazy looking back. I saw 80% of the gains over the last year. Once I met with Don and changed my eating habits, I've been able to keep my healthy weight long-term, not just for a few months like my other "diet" efforts in the past. I've gained and lost 20+ pounds multiple times and I realized that you must really embrace the nutrition portion along with exercise to meet your fitness goals. Don, thanks again for your help, knowledge and motivation." ~ **Jeremy Padgett, client and Fit 24/7 gym member**

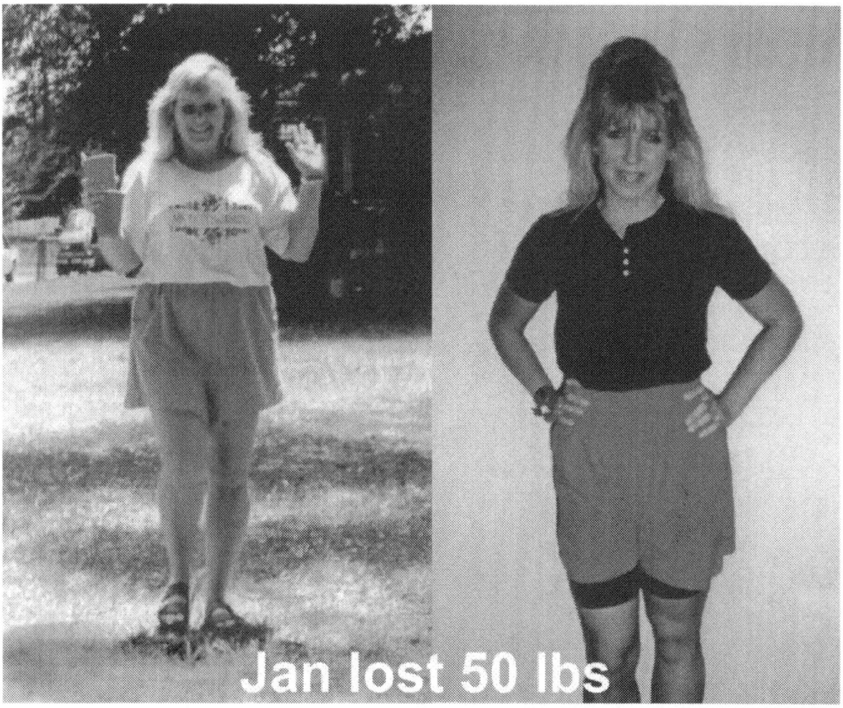

"Though it has been just over twenty years that I started training with Don, I still feel such gratitude and respect for him for keeping me motivated and encouraged to have accomplished one of the greatest challenges of my life. But what we did in less than a year was way more than me losing 50 pounds, it was the beginning of realizing just how important my happiness, health, and wellness are! I am truly blessed to have trained with an incredible, honest, genuine, hard- working, and dedicated fitness coach who I will always consider my friend. Thank you, Don for leaving a lasting impression on all who have been fortunate enough to have had the kind of opportunity like I did." ~ **Jan Hilger, client and Fit 24/7 gym member**

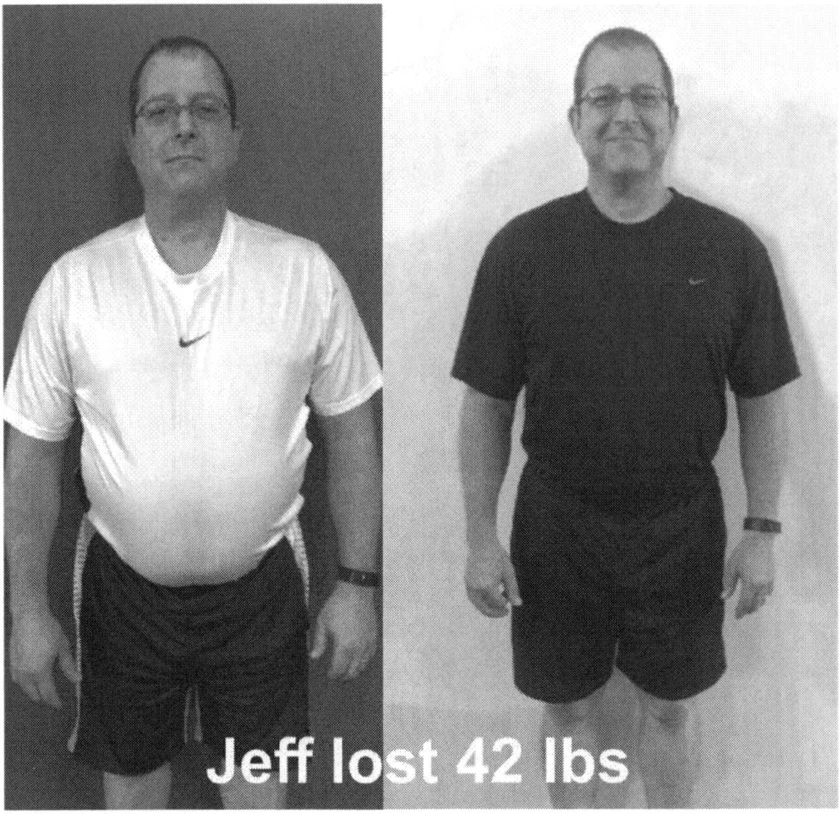

"I lost 41 pounds in 8 weeks on Don's weight training program and eating Plan. Needless to say, it works!" **~ Jeff Titus, client and Fit 24/7 gym member**

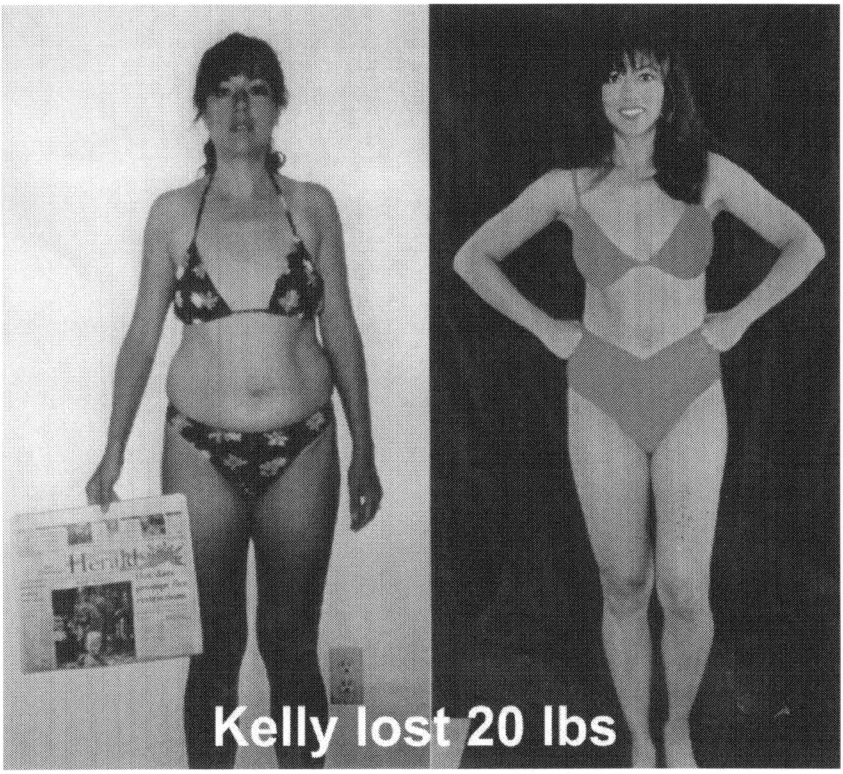

"The concept of exercise was very foreign to me because it had never been a part of my life. I was not an athletic person, so I felt very shy about working out around others. Don became my guru. He took the information he learned and used it to customize a fitness and diet program I could actually do. It fit my personality, my lifestyle, my schedule... It fit ME. I literally transformed myself in 12 weeks. It was an amazing experience having strangers at the gym approach me and tell me I inspired them by seeing my progress. It was kind of a magical time in my life that I will never forget. Nor will I ever forget Don and his plethora of information, wisdom, and guidance. **~ Kelly Mitchell, client and Fit 24/7 gym member**

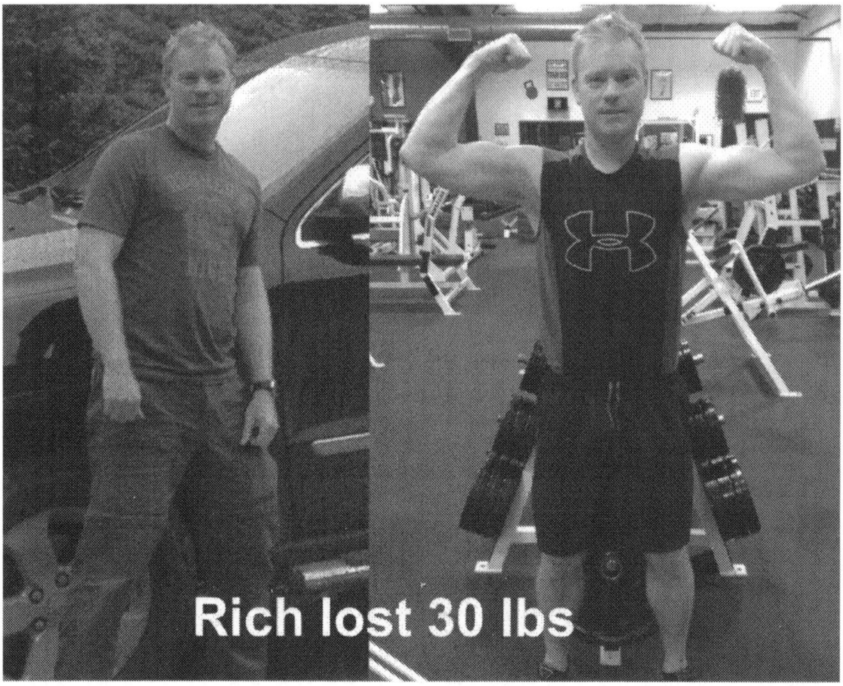

"Don's expertly designed programs are uncomplicated to sustain and have provided me with the tools to be in the best shape of my life. In six months, I lost 30 pounds!"
~ Rich Millard, client and Fit 24/7 gym member

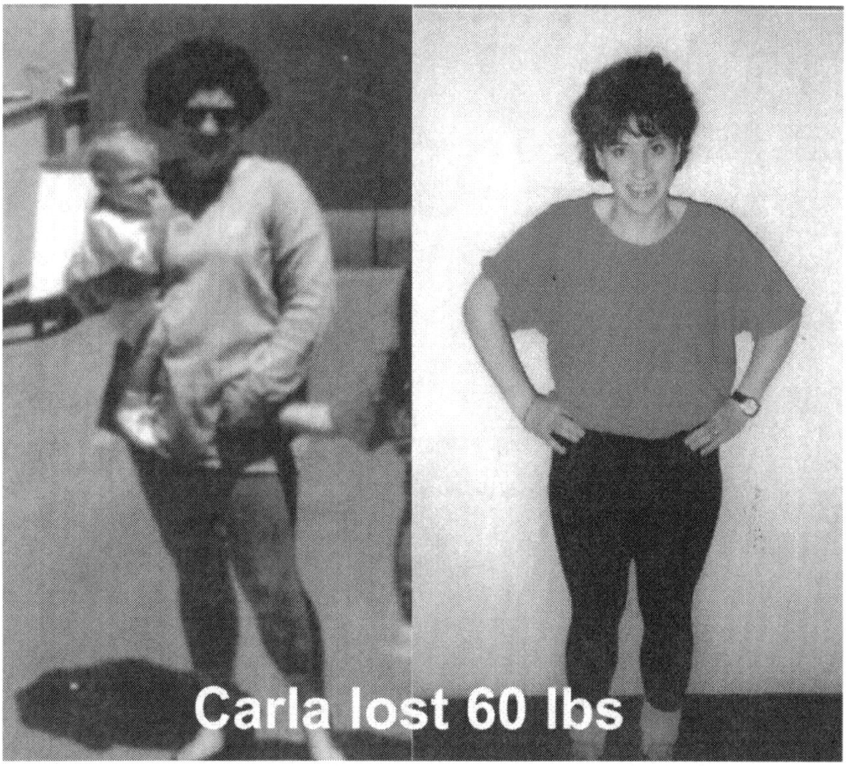

"Following Don's training program and eating plan, I lost an amazing 60 pounds in less than a year!" ~ **Carla Wright, client and Fit 24/7 gym member**

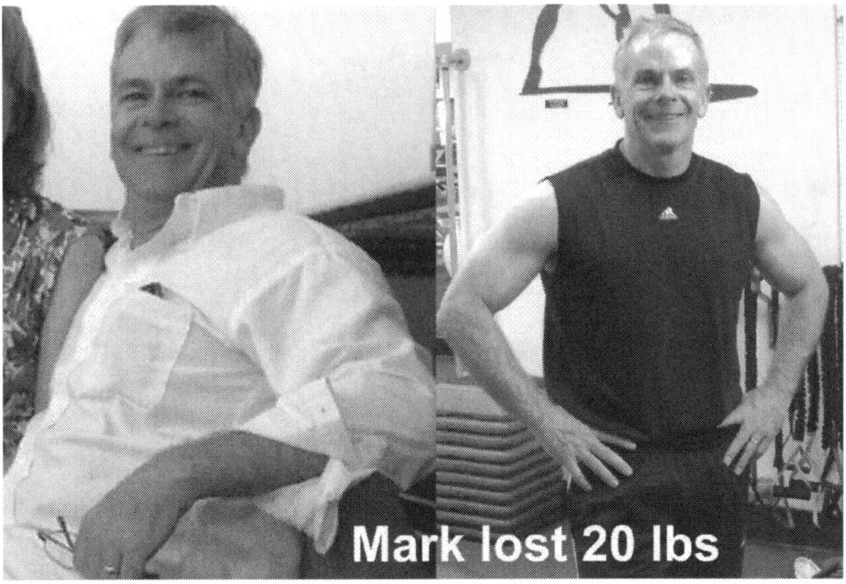

"I like seeing a more fit looking guy in the mirror, instead of an old flabby looking guy that was there three months ago, and my wife is proud of me, and working out more regularly herself. Don's plans are well thought out, produce results, motivation, and are achievable. I encourage anyone who wants to get stronger, leaner, look better, and feel more confident and proud of themselves, to meet with Don, make a plan, and get after it!" ~ **Mark Walters, client and Fit 24/7 gym member**

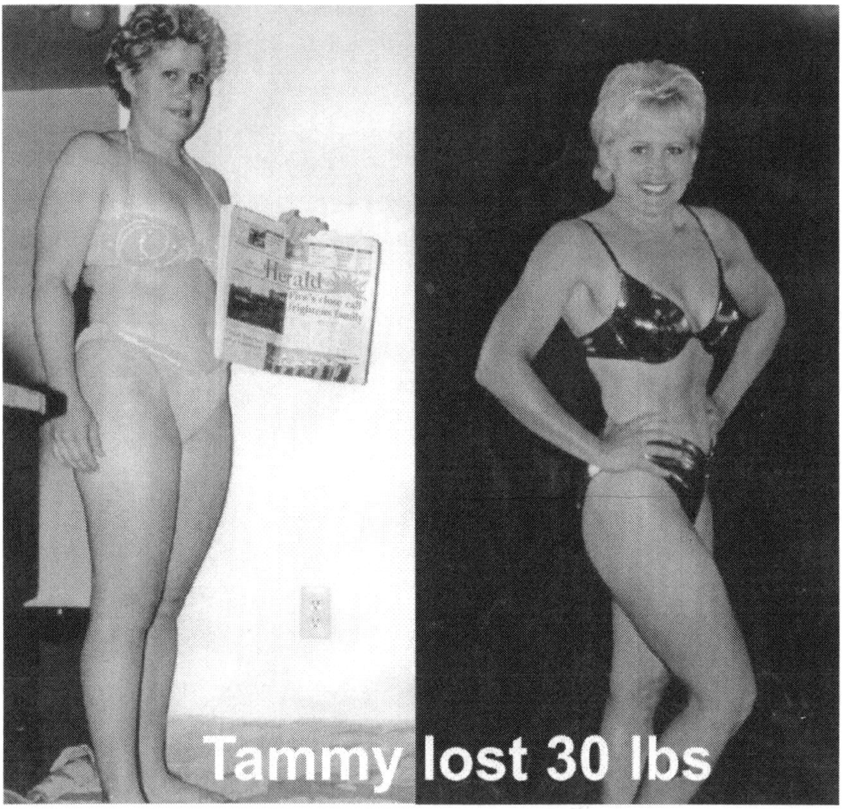

"Don's programs helped me lose 30 pounds in just 12 weeks! I feel like a different person." ~ **Tammy Wyatt, client and Fit 24/7 gym member**

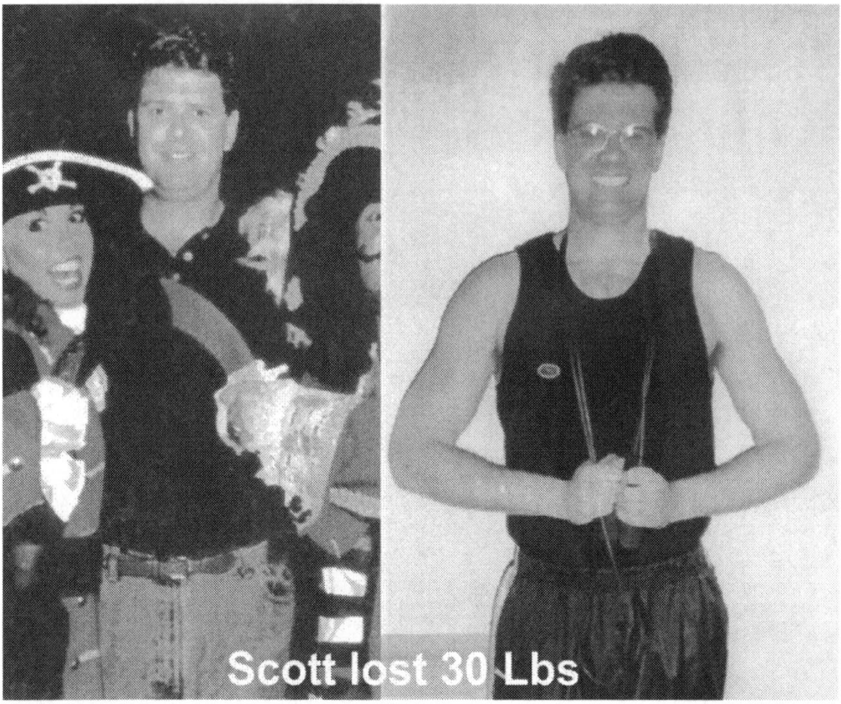

"In the first month, I lost 12 honest pounds. My energy skyrocketed, and my self-esteem started to rise as well. Three months later, I had gone from 208 lbs. to 176 lbs., and I am a completely different person. I have noticed muscles and veins I thought were only achievable in the movies or in a select dedicated few." ~ **Scott Mason, client and Fit 24/7 gym member**

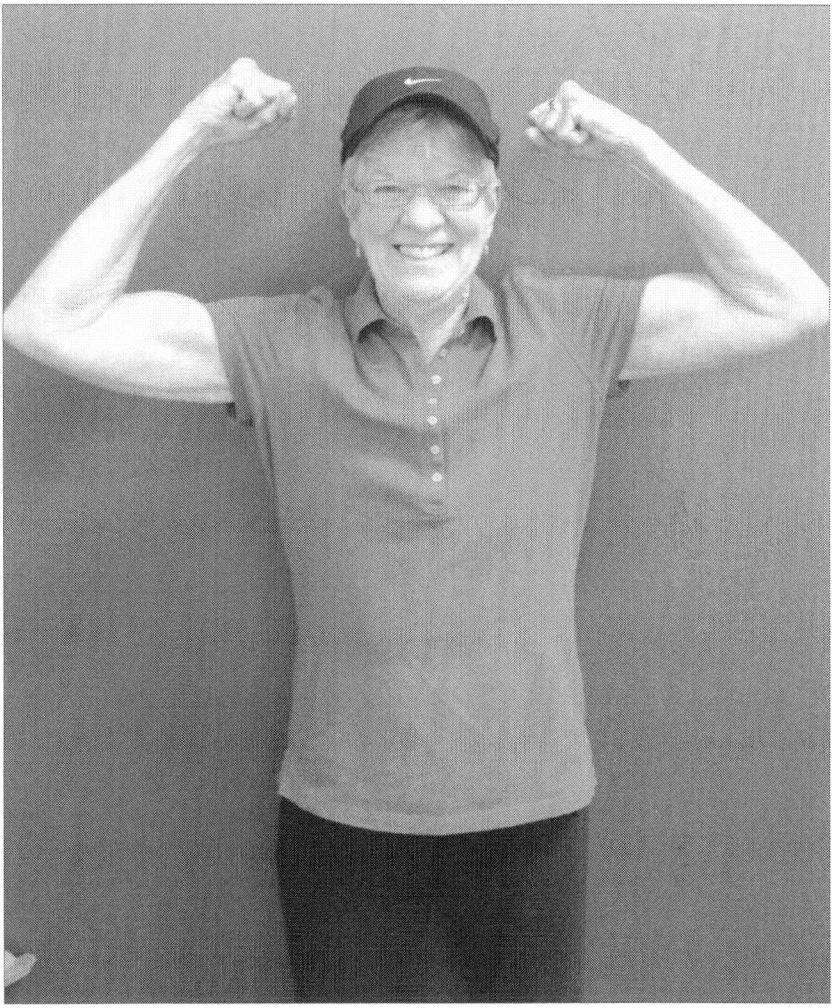

"Never in my wildest dreams did I think that I would develop arm muscles at 70 years old, but I did. Wow! Real muscles! Thank you Don, for helping to add a new dimension to my life. Let's all keep moving!" ~ **Client and Fit 24/7 gym member, the late Linda Allenbaugh**

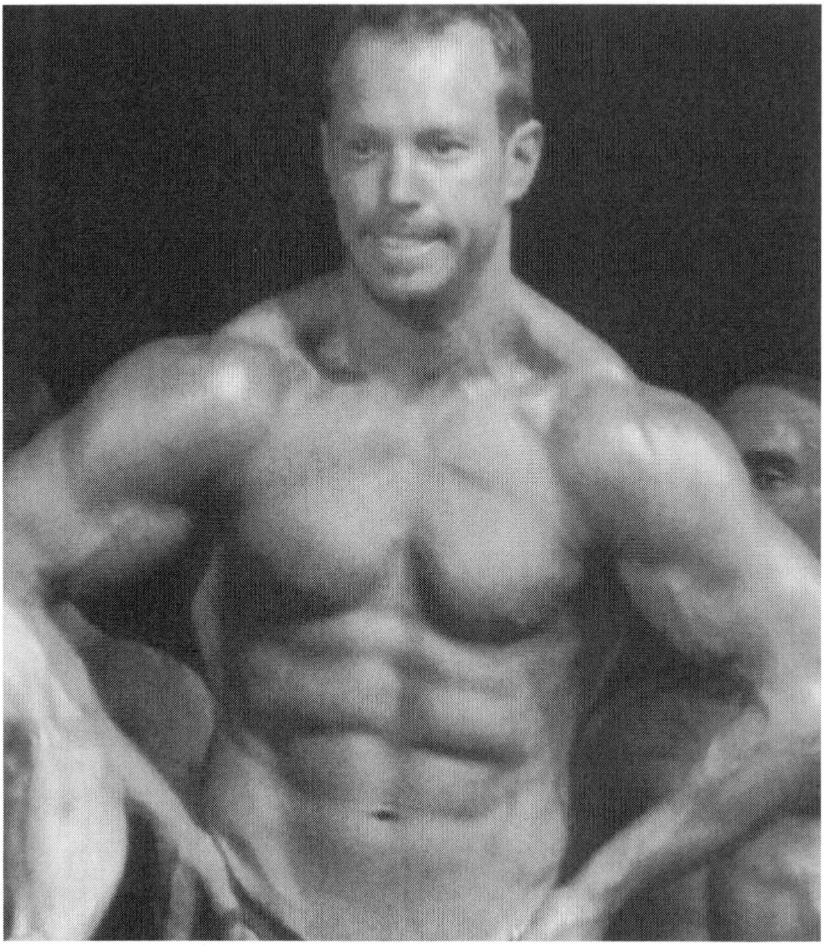

"Don helped me to line up specific nutrition and workout regimens with timelines to help me attain my goals for a bodybuilding competition. With Don's help, I was able to increase my muscle size while decreasing my body fat percentage. During the final eight weeks of training, I was able to lose 8+ pounds of fat, while maintaining my lean muscle. On competition day, I was truly impressed with my transformation. Thanks Don!" ~ **Michael Testa, client and Fit 24/7 gym member**

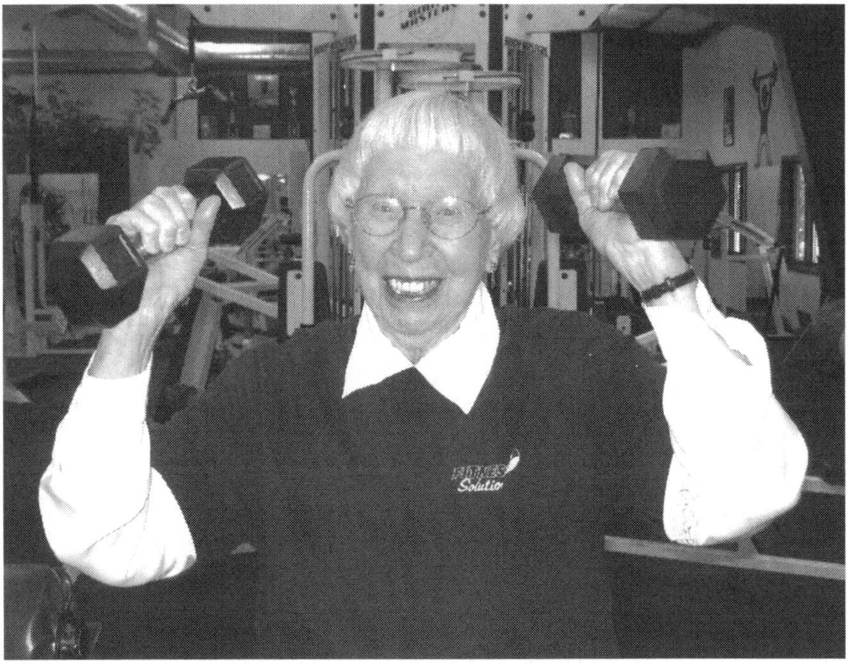

"Over time, I lost the strength in my legs to such a degree that I couldn't step into my son's vehicle. After three months in Don's gym, there was a phenomenal difference. At 92 years old, I no longer needed assistance. I depend on an every-other-day routine." ~ **Fit 24/7 gym member, the late Lorena Nash**

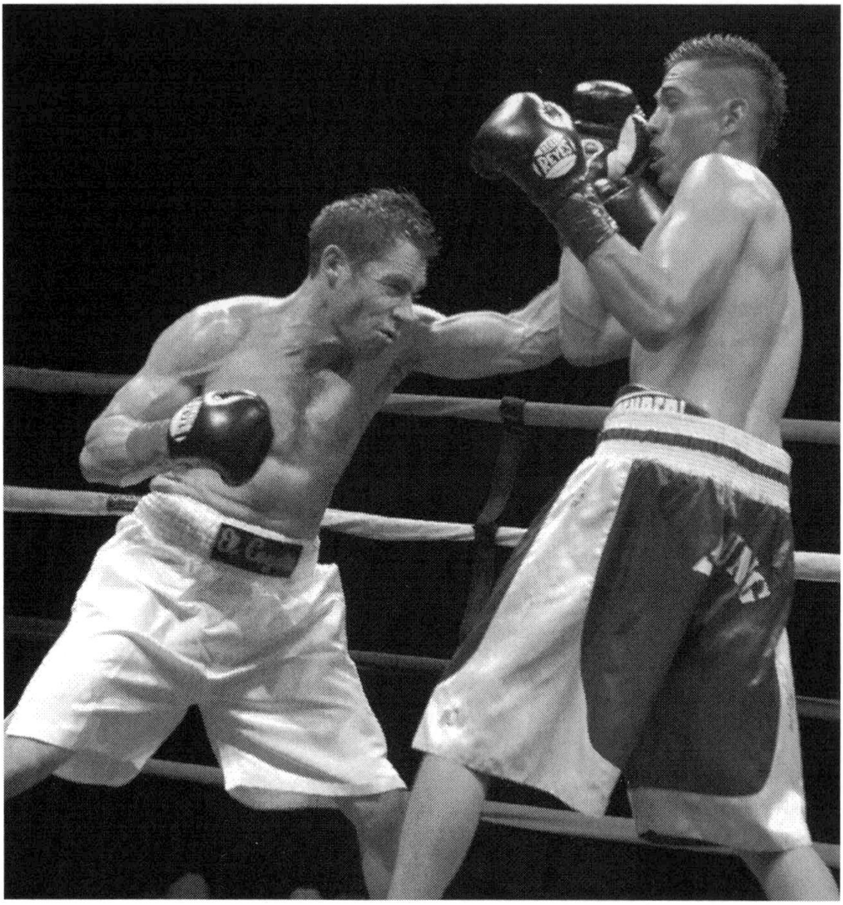

"Don, thanks for the support, along with the reminder, to always maintain a positive outlook on things." **~ Miguel "El Coyote" Gallegos, professional boxer and Fit 24/7 gym member**

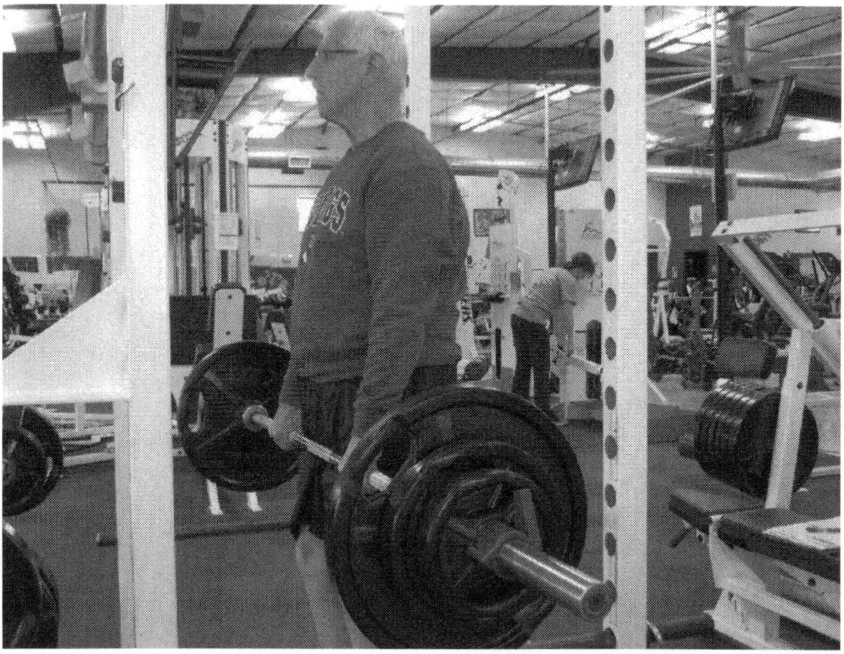

"I've watched Don work with clients for 15 years now and he never seems to sluff-off. His clients are very important to him. Now that I'm one of those clients, he's important to me. At 75 years old and battling Parkinson's disease, I'm still pulling over 200 pounds off the rack. In 1987, at 46 years old and weighing 275 pounds, I was the USPF National Powerlifting Champion: bench-440; squat-573; deadlift-589."
~ Close friend, client and Fit 24/7 gym member, the late Tony Teets

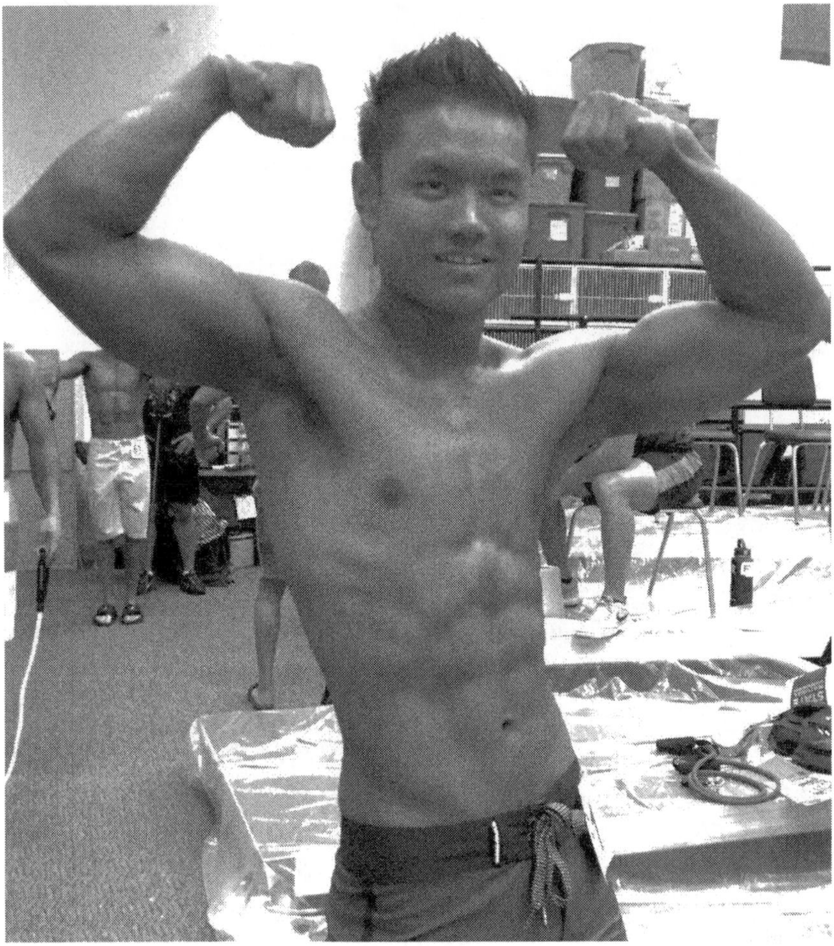

"Don not only provided me a great workout routine and diet, he gave me a new way of thinking when it comes to bodybuilding, which is always evolving with a learning mindset. It's not a goal, it's a lifestyle. My advice to anybody is, face yourself and be honest - that's when progress happens." ~ **Kenjok Bhotia, client and Fit 24/7 gym member, amateur physique competitor**

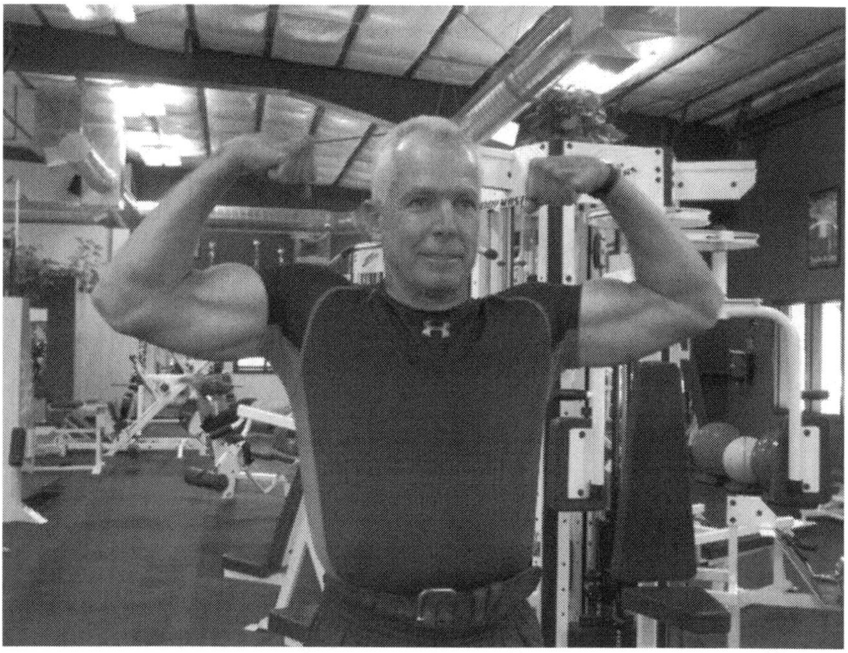

"Don is passionate about his gym and his clientele's health and fitness. He regularly holds classes on training methods and nutrition. It is like a family affair. He shows interest in everyone's well-being and always makes time to talk to you about health and fitness. Following many of Don's nutrition recommendations has made a significant improvement in both mine and my wife's fitness. My wife is 66 years old and I am 71. Neither of us take any medications and we live active healthy lives. Finding Don and his gym has been a true blessing in our lives." ~ **Ken Nash, Fit 24/7 gym member**

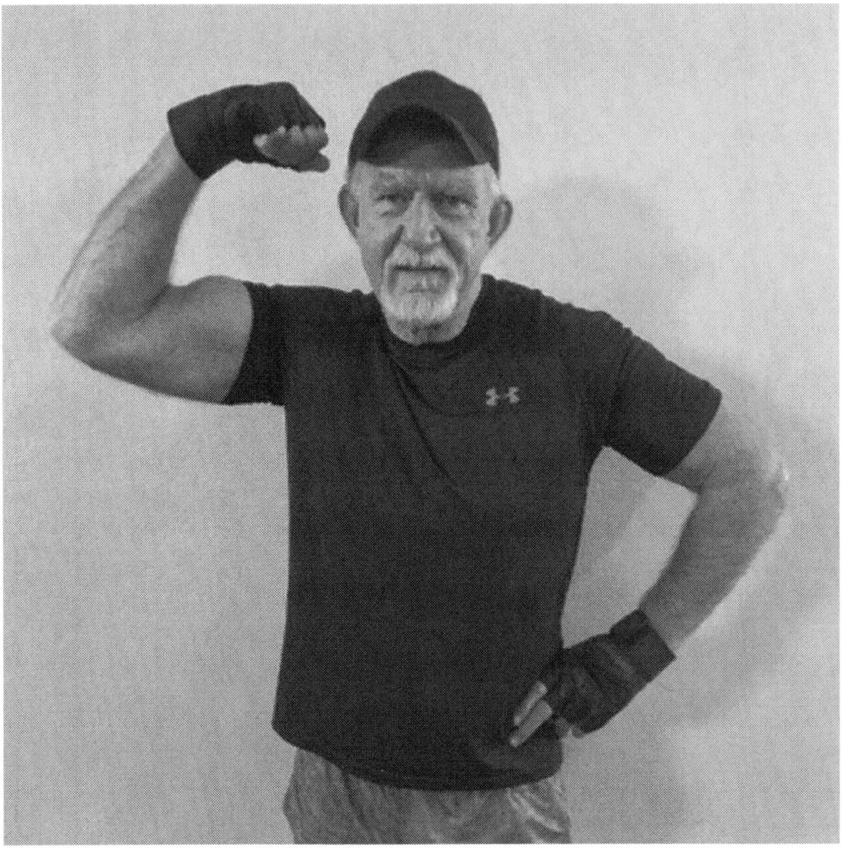

"I had worked out for most of my life with okay results. It wasn't until Don counseled me on good nutrition, consistency, and a balanced and varied workout routine, that I made progress. I went from nearly 250 pounds to a steady 190 pounds and have gained strength and stamina. At 65, I am stronger than I was in my 30s and 40s, pressing 100-pound dumbbells for 10 repetitions. Recently, I did 1,000 pushups in one afternoon just to test myself."
~ Kayo Folsom, Fit 24/7 gym member

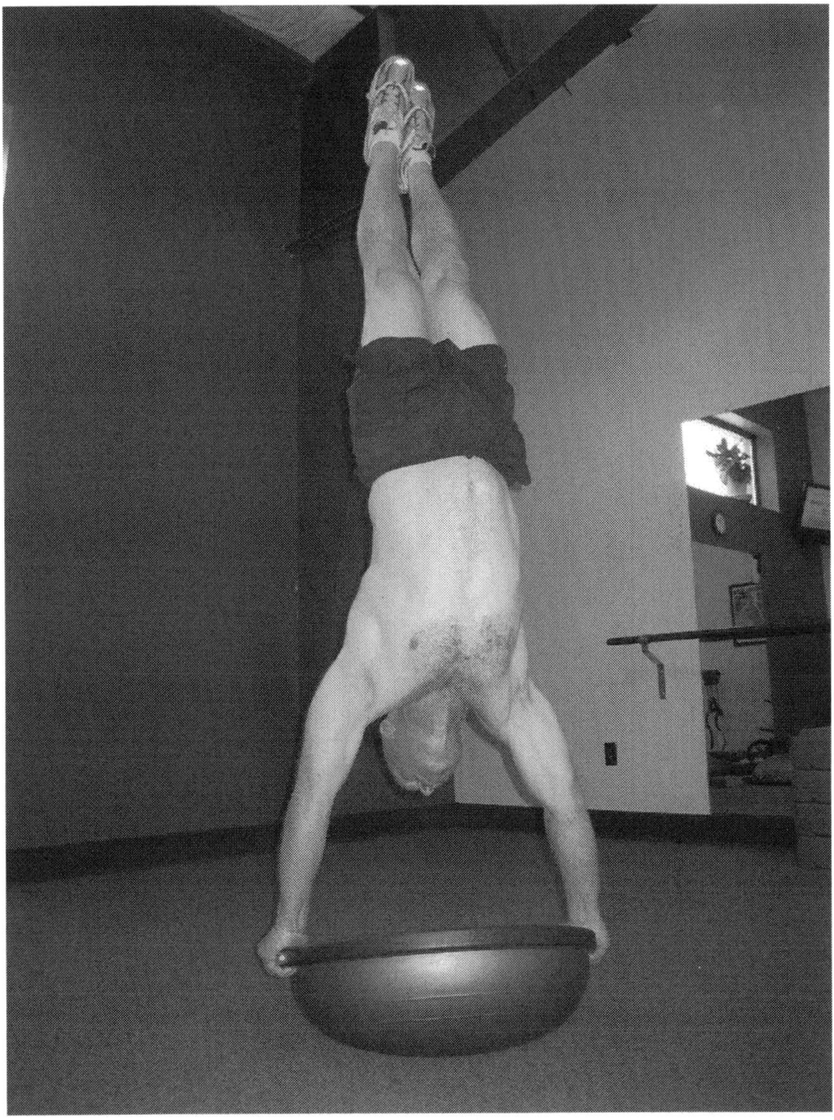

"Thanks Don for your knowledge and input on proper foods and life balance for a strong and lean body. At 49 years old, I used Don's diet and workout ideas to finish 2nd in my class at the first bodybuilding competition I entered."
~ Randy Gerken, Fit 24/7 gym member

Don's Clients: Other Testimonials

"Thank you so much for giving me the tools to make my life 100% better! I considered myself crippled, and my doctor told me I needed both knees replaced. Even after surgeries, I still walked with a limp and they were swollen and painful all the time. When you introduced me to your eating plan and training program, you told me the diet would help take away inflammation out of my joints. What an understatement! It made a huge difference in my knees in just a few weeks. I have gone from a size 16 to a size 12 in about two months. I did not think it was possible to get this kind of improvement!" ~ **Diane Steinbacher, client and Fit 24/7 gym member**

"My weight had previously bounced up and down despite a balanced, healthy (or so I thought) diet, and a rigorous three-day-a-week exercise routine. I even quit drinking beer (gasp!) thinking that might help. Still unable to reduce my weight, I contacted Don. His brief, but informative eating plan laid out the why and wherefore that has enabled me to reach my target. I went from 188 pounds to 170 pounds in three months. What is most astonishing is that it's an eating plan that I really enjoy and will have no difficulty continuing." ~ **Paul Conrady, client and Fit 24/7 gym member**

"I was very skeptical. I have tried many weight-loss plans, with all ending in failure. To my surprise, Don's plan was easy to follow and I didn't feel hungry. I lost 15 pounds in 2 months. This is a miracle for me!" ~ **Jeanne Zeman, client and Fit 24/7 gym member**

"In the time I have trained with Don, I have lost over 35 pounds, dramatically changed my muscle-to-fat ratio, improved my cardiovascular performance by over 20%, and most importantly, I enjoy my training time with him." **~ Richard Cortese, client and Fit 24/7 gym member**

"I started working out with Don in my early fifties as my body was going through all sorts of changes. Don has instructed me, monitored me, educated me, and more importantly, cared for my well-being. I can without a doubt, state that as I approach 70, I would not have the life force or strong capable body without Don's tutelage and care. Working with Don on a weekly basis has definitely improved my quality of life." **~ Christy Pollard, client and Fit 24/7 gym member**

"By following Don's customized eating plan and workout program, I lost 10 pounds in the first month and went from 185 to 163 pounds overall. At 36, I am in the best shape of my life! Do yourself a life-changing favor and schedule a meeting to discuss his eating plan. It will be one of the best investments you ever make!" **~ Trey Brunson, client and Fit 24/7 gym member**

"Don's Bell^3 Weight Training Program is amazing! As a 40 year old woman, I didn't expect to see that level of strength. I highly recommend it for women and men of all ages and fitness levels. His exceptional training and nutrition guidance helped me build muscle and strength quickly." **~ Katie Knox, client and Fit 24/7 gym member**

"Your workout and diet program helped me win the 2001 Overall World Championship of Cowboy Action Shooting." **~ Gene Pearcy, client and Fit 24/7 gym member**

"Don provided me with accurate information about how to train and how to eat for overall good health. The extra weight is gone and has stayed gone, yeah! But, the real benefits are increased energy, strength, and a total body image. Instead of battling genetics and aging, I am truly enjoying a new lifestyle!" ~ **Candace Alburn, client and Fit 24/7 gym member**

"I have used Don's eating plan and have had terrific results. I went from 223 to 195 pounds in just a few months. I have also used Don's personal training and look pretty good for a great grandfather." ~ **Tom Minnich, client and Fit 24/7 gym member**

"Working with Don helped me completely restructure my workouts to focus on major muscle groups that burn more calories. Thanks to only two 30-45 minute workouts a week for three months, I have been able to lose 12 pounds and greatly increase my strength and endurance in other activities. I'm stronger and faster than I have ever been mountain biking and can't wait to use my new and improved body skiing this winter!" ~ **Dr Kiley Berry, client and Fit 24/7 gym member**

"Don designed a leg workout specifically for my bicycling and the results were phenomenal! At 55 years old and a bodyweight of 170 pounds, I was squatting up to 250 pounds." ~ **Les Johnson, client and Fit 24/7 gym member**

"First of all, I hate working out! However, Don has given me workouts that don't let me cheat and that work. His Bell3 workout plans have definitely made a difference in how I look and feel." ~ **Kathy Coutlee, client and Fit 24/7 gym member**

"I would turn to food and eat to comfort my anxieties. By following Don's advice, I really started to see food differently. Comfort and convenience gave way to health and vitality. By the second week into Don's eating plan, I lost all junk food cravings. I lost 32 pounds in just four months." **~ Keith Cramer, client and Fit 24/7 gym member**

"I had been training with weights for over ten years with minimal results. During the year I had Don's guidance in eating and working out, I gained the knowledge to help me be in the best shape of my life. His style makes individuals feel comfortable, no matter what level they are at. I lost 25 pounds in six months (220-195). My body fat went from 27% to 17% and my strength soared on all my lifts." **~ Chad Midkiff, client and Fit 24/7 gym member**

"I met with Don while visiting Durango concerning weight loss. I am 61 years old and went from 203 pounds to 183 pounds in 8 weeks. Thanks, Don." **~ Judge Don Barnett, client and Fit 24/7 gym member**

"When I look back at my 35 plus years of weight training, Don has provided me with a wealth of knowledge. Because of him, I am always open-minded to new training philosophies and techniques. My biggest changes occurred when he educated me on proper nutrition, specifically what type, how much, and when macronutrients (carbs, protein, and fat) should be consumed. I would not have achieved my goal of competing in a bodybuilding contest without his support. I lost 26 pounds (180-154) in 16 weeks and was awarded 1st place in the 2007 NPC Natural Colorado (Men's Open Lightweight Division)." **~ Damian Arellano, lifelong friend**

Don's Bodybuilding Photos

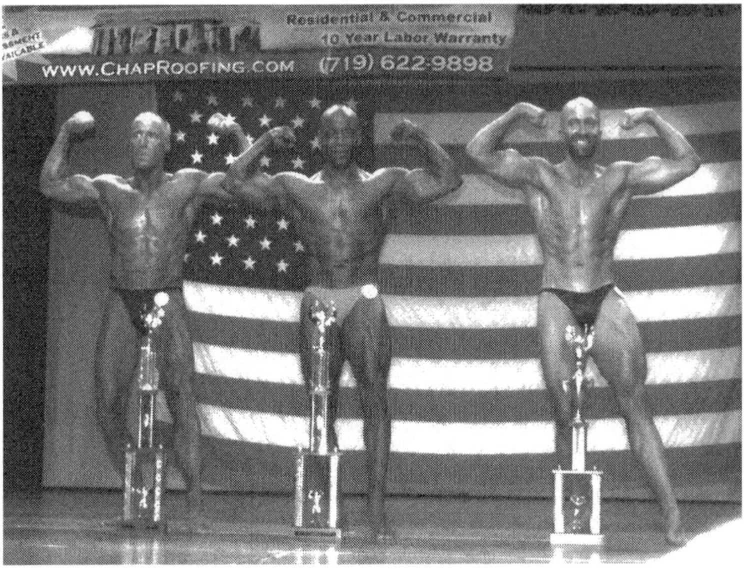

2007 Colorado Armed Forces

Natural Bodybuilding Contest -Masters Class

Don (far right) placed 3rd

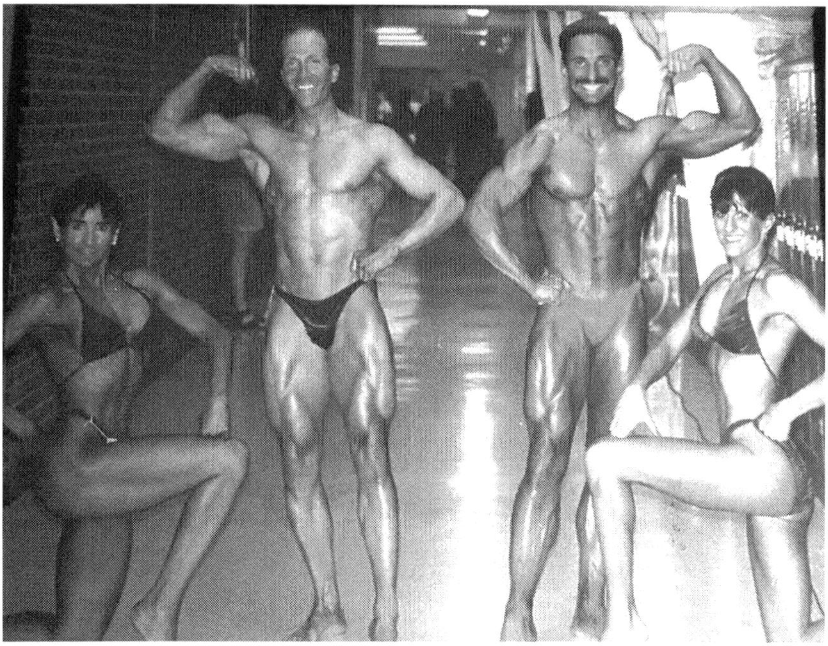

1996 Colorado Natural Bodybuilding Championships

Don (2nd from left) placed 5th

His wife Teri (far right) placed 3rd

Section Three

Nutrition Myths and Facts

Weight gain and weight loss is all about calories in and calories out.

Myth.

Since the 1920s, we have been told that calorie counting is the key to losing weight. Calories became the most important tool in the fight to lose weight. Calorie counting promised a scientific and foolproof method of weight loss. *Calorie* is a French-derived term indicating a "unit of heat," with *caloric* meaning a fluid believed to embody heat. Caloric faded as a theory, but calorie became indispensable in the study of energy and heat in engines and later in humans as part of metabolic and food studies. Before becoming a thing of fashion, the calorie had a less glamorous role in agriculture, factories, and laboratories. By the end of the 1920s, the calorie was a constant feature of the American diet, and has stuck ever since, for better or worse.

Calories do matter, but hormones matter more. Hormones have a greater effect on cravings, hunger, metabolism, mood, and energy; the caloric number of food means nothing to the body. Man-made foods like bread, cereal, flavored yogurt, soda, pasta, sweets, etc., are absorbed quickly into the bloodstream because of their lack of important macronutrients. Protein, fat, and fiber, as well as the micronutrient vitamins, minerals, and antioxidants, are all critical elements for the body. Eating food that is absent of these vital nutrients will cause chemical reactions to occur, which sabotages our ability to lose fat.

Specifically, in response to the consumption of nutrient poor foods, the pancreas sends a surge of insulin into the bloodstream. A bit of insulin is used, but the rest goes to fat storage. Next, our brain gets a boost of serotonin, which can make us feel good at first, but the excess serotonin converts to tryptophan (best known as an ingredient in turkey) and makes us tired soon thereafter. Then, the brain releases ghrelin, making us hungry. High sugar and high flour foods make us gain excess fat, feel tired, get hangry (hungry and angry), and feel unsatisfied because bad chemicals (hormones) flood our system. These foods are really *anti-*nutrients, increasing the U.S. epidemic of numerous diseases: obesity, heart disease, diabetes, cancer, arthritis, and more.

On the other hand, what happens when we eat foods of the earth: eggs, nuts, seeds, meats, fish, vegetables, etc.? These are the foods that we were intended to eat, the stuff that has allowed us to flourish as a species for thousands of years. The protein, fat, and fiber, as well as numerous vitamins, minerals, and antioxidants found in these natural foods are what our bodies want and need. Here, we see an entirely different chemical reaction. Instead of releasing insulin into the bloodstream, the pancreas now secretes glucagon (not to be confused with glycogen). Glucagon is a fat burning hormone. Dopamine is released from the brain, making us alert. And instead of ghrelin making us hungry, leptin is released, making us feel satiated. Now, we are on a path of becoming lean, alert, and satisfied, as well as decreasing our risk of the many aforementioned diseases.

Something to chew on: A pancake (depending on the size) and an egg have the same calories, about 70; a jelly donut and a chicken thigh are equal at about 270 calories. Which foods will make you fat, feel tired, and hungry? Which ones will make you lean, alert, and satisfied? Eating 2,000 calories a day from cereal, juice, and bread won't give you the same mental and physical results as eating eggs, meat, nuts and vegetables. That said, eating an excess of calories over time will cause you to gain weight. However, my recommendation is that you focus on eating whole foods that are rich in nutrition and give less thought to counting calories.

Get advice from a nutritional counselor who understands hormones.

"Food is the most abused anxiety drug."
~ Unknown

If you have high cholesterol, you have heart disease.

Myth.

For decades, cholesterol has been a highly publicized scapegoat, identified as the primary cause of heart disease. However, cholesterol itself is not the culprit. Turns out that the biggest factor in an individual's cholesterol level is not diet, but genetics or heredity. Cholesterol is a soft, white, waxy substance found in every cell in your body and is necessary to produce cell membranes, hormones, Vitamin D, bile acids, and more. The human liver is designed to remove excess cholesterol from the body, but genetics play the largest part in the liver's *ability* to regulate cholesterol to a healthy level.

There are two types of cholesterol: High-density lipoprotein HDL ("good" cholesterol), which helps keep cholesterol away from your arteries and removes excess arterial plaque, helping prevent heart disease. The other is low-density lipoprotein LDL ("bad" cholesterol), which may build up in your arteries and form plaque. Plaque narrows your arteries and also might break off as a clot, which may go to your heart or brain and cause a heart attack or stroke. But, total cholesterol level is not a good indicator in determining your risk of heart disease, unless it is above 330 mg/dL. Unfortunately, the American Heart Association (AHA) recommends a total cholesterol of 200 mg/dl. This is the sum of your blood's cholesterol content, including HDL, LDLs, and very low-density lipoprotein (VLDLs). It is misleading when they combine these three types.

Also making up your cholesterol count is Triglyceride (elevated levels of this dangerous fat may lead to diabetes and heart disease). The National Cholesterol Education Program sets guidelines for triglyceride levels: Normal = less than 150 milligrams per deciliter; Borderline high = 150-199; High = 200-499. Another substance is lipoprotein(a) or Lp(a), which is made up of an LDL cholesterol plus a protein (apoprotein a). High levels of this may also increase your risk of heart disease. A good indicator of heart disease risk is your Triglyceride-to-HDL ratio. To determine this, divide your triglycerides by your HDL level. The ideal ratio is 2 or below.

To combat high cholesterol levels, many doctors prescribe statins to their patients (one in four Americans ages 45 and older take statins). However, more than 900 studies now prove that statins can have adverse, even deadly, side effects, including increased cancer risk, sexual dysfunction, diabetes, cognitive loss, and muscle weakness.

The only people who might benefit from statins are those with familial hypercholesterolemia, which is a genetic defect that makes a person resistant to traditional measures of normalizing cholesterol.

Statin use causes a depletion of Coenzyme Q10 (CoQ10), a cofactor essential for the creation of ATP (adenosine triphosphate) molecules needed for cellular energy production. Low levels of CoQ10 may lead to fatigue, soreness, muscle weakness, and heart failure!

Here are tips for protecting your heart without drugs:

- Exercise regularly
- Minimize stress levels

- Minimize alcohol consumption
- Add fermented foods to your diet
- Avoid smoking and chewing tobacco
- Eat a lot of raw food (salads, nuts, etc.)
- Get seven-to-nine hours of quality sleep per night
- Minimize sugars and grains in your diet, including juice
- Consume lots of Omega-3 fatty acids (salmon, fish oil, flaxseed oil, grass-fed beef)
- Get plenty of sun exposure without sunscreen (15-20 minutes a day) to optimize your Vitamin D levels
- Replace synthetic trans fats and harmful vegetable oils with healthy fats

In 2012, Dr. Dwight Lundell, MD, wrote in his book, *Prevent Disease*:

"Today is my day to right a wrong with medical and scientific fact. I trained for 25-years with prominent physicians labeled 'opinion makers.' We insisted heart disease resulted from the simple fact of elevated blood cholesterol. Prescribing medications to lower cholesterol and diets low in fat was standard. Neither are scientifically or morally defensible. More Americans will die of heart disease this year than ever before. It is the number #1 cause of death in the U.S. Without inflammation present, there is no way that cholesterol would accumulate in the blood vessel wall and cause heart disease or stroke. Without inflammation, cholesterol would move freely through the body as nature intended. Inflammation causes cholesterol to be trapped. Toxins and foods the body was never designed to process cause chronic inflammation. These toxins and foods lead to heart disease, stroke, diabetes, and obesity. Highly processed carbs are the biggest culprit (sugar, flour, and all products made from them) and excess omega 6 oils like soybean, corn, and sunflower oils that are found in them. These foods have been the mainstay of the American diet for 60-years. These foods are slowly poisoning everyone. Of my 5000+ clients spanning 25-years, all share one common denominator, inflammation of the arteries."

Seventy-five-percent of the cholesterol in your body is made by your liver. Only 25% comes from the foods you eat. Many of the healthiest foods on the planet happen to be rich in cholesterol: eggs, grass-fed beef, and butter, just to name a few.

Twenty-five-percent of the cholesterol in your body is found in your brain where it plays critically important roles. In the brain, cholesterol aids membrane function, acts as an antioxidant, and serves as the raw material from which we make testosterone, progesterone, estrogen, cortisol, and vitamin D. Research shows that in the elderly, those with the best memory function have the highest levels of cholesterol. Low cholesterol is associated with increased risk of depression and even death.

Because of big pharma's power in selling cholesterol lowering medications and the media touting the benefits of those drugs, many doctors still recommend that people avoid foods high in cholesterol, like shrimp, eggs, etc., when these dietary changes have minimal effect on lowering cholesterol.

"If you're afraid of butter, use cream." ~ **Julia Child, American chef, author and television personality**

Consuming saturated fat is healthy.

Fact.

Even though we have been told for decades that saturated fat causes heart disease, it has never been proven. Go back to flawed research from the 1950s when a guy named Ancel Keys, a University of Minnesota physiologist, published a paper (*Seven Countries Study*) that blamed dietary fat intake for the increase of heart disease. There were major flaws in his study, as he only used data from a small portion of the countries involved in the original study (7 out of 22). Not coincidentally, these seven countries just so happened to be the only countries providing funding for the study. Countries were eliminated when they didn't want to fund the research. The French and Germans, who were originally part of the study, but later eliminated, showed relatively low rates of heart disease even though they were living on a diet rich in saturated fats.

For thousands of years, our ancestors survived and thrived on saturated fats from meat, eggs, and dairy. The bulk of their diet was saturated fat and protein. Current research on various peoples around the world, i.e.: Abkhazia (Azerbaijan), Hunza (Tibet), and Masai (Africa) whose diets are high in saturated animal fats, demonstrate very few diseases and an incredibly high life expectancy.

A sizeable recent study following 135,335 people in 18 countries and five continents, which was published in 2017 in *The Lancet*, a renowned, peer-reviewed medical journal, shows that eating fat *lowers* the risk of mortality. Further, the study showed that the type of fat didn't have any bearing on the risk of heart disease. Saturated fat consumption was inversely related to strokes. Those eating high-carb diets had a nearly 30-percent higher death rate than those eating low-carb diets. Meanwhile, those eating high-fat diets had a 23-percent lower death rate during the study period.

A 2010 study published in the *American Journal of Clinical Nutrition* showed that "there is no significant evidence for concluding that dietary saturated fat is associated with an increased risk of coronary heart disease."

In addition, the National Institute of Health funded a multi-million dollar study known as the Women's Health Initiative (WHI). One of the three parts to this in-depth research was the Dietary Modification Trial. This multi-year study (1993 - 2005) tracked over 48,000 women aged 50-79 years old. The subjects were put on a low-fat diet for the entire time. The study, which is the largest ever of its type, showed no significant difference in risks of heart disease, stroke, breast cancer, or colon cancer compared to those eating normal amounts of dietary fat, including saturated fat.

The benefits of saturated fat include:

- Nutritious
- Tastes amazing
- Good for weight loss
- Increased HDL levels
- Vital for our bone health
- Antimicrobial properties
- Tolerates high heat as a cooking fat
- Gives cell membranes stiffness and integrity
- Constitutes at least 50% of the cell membranes

- Protects against harmful microorganisms in the digestive tract

The idea that saturated fats cause heart disease is completely wrong, but the statement has been published so many times over decades that it is difficult to convince people otherwise, unless they are willing to take the time to read and learn what produced the anti-saturated fat agenda.

"Even though the focus of dietary recommendations is usually a reduction of saturated fat intake, no relation between saturated fat and a risk of coronary heart disease was observed in the most informative studies to date," writes Dr. Walter Willett, Professor of Nutritional Epidemiology, Harvard Medical School.

"Saturated fats are the preferred fats for the heart, carriers for fat soluble vitamins (A, D, E and K) and useful in lowering cholesterol levels (palmitic and stearic acids). They are effective as anti-plaque and antifungal agents as well (lauric acid)," notes Dr. Joseph Mercola, an alternative medicine proponent and osteopathic physician.

The best sources of saturated fat are eggs, naturally raised meats, butter (from grass-fed cows), coconut oil, avocados, nuts, and seeds.

"One cannot think, love, or sleep well if one has not dined well."
~ Virginia Woolf, 20th century English writer

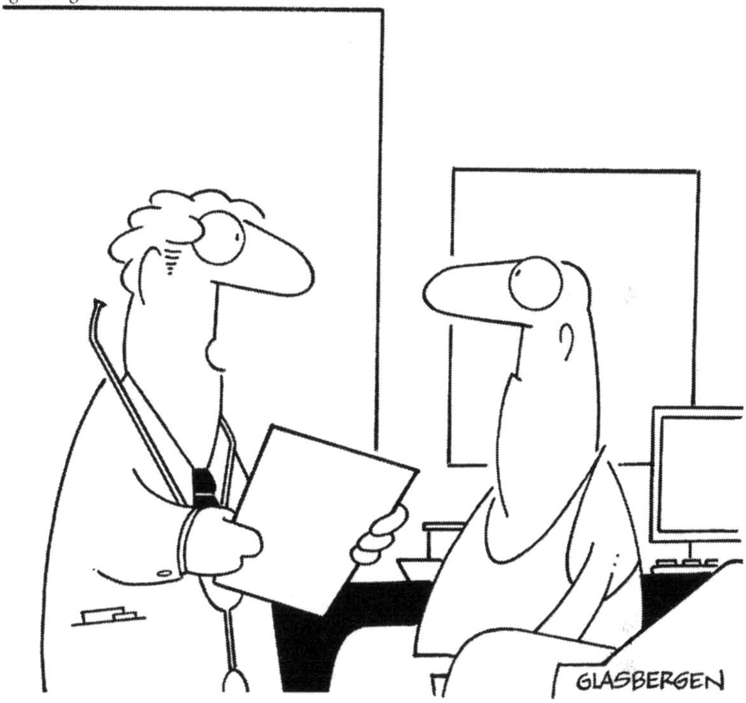

"The good news, it's OK to eat butter after all. The bad news, it's not OK to eat any of the things you like to put butter on."

All carbohydrates are absorbed quickly and convert into fat.

Myth.

Along with protein and fat, carbohydrates are one of the three macronutrients that provide fuel for the body. While many carbohydrates are bad for us (sugar, refined flour, etc.), there are many that are very healthy. The best carbohydrate choices are ones that are moderate to high in fiber (10-20 grams per cup) and are therefore absorbed slowly (indicated by a low glycemic index (1-55), These carbs give us prolonged energy, control hunger, and aid in weight loss and weight maintenance.

Examples of good carbs are most vegetables (except corn and some root veggies, which tend to be moderate-to-high glycemic), nuts, seeds, legumes, quinoa, oats (slow cooked and unsweetened), wild rice, brown rice, sweet potatoes, and some fruits like apples, berries, grapes, oranges, peaches, pears, and plums.

Good carbohydrates provide many benefits:

- **Cellular recognition** - Improve our immune system
- **Fat oxidation** - Carbs break down into oxaloacetic acid, which metabolizes fats
- **G.I. function** - Help calcium absorption and bone health
- **Flavor** - More varieties than fat and protein
- **Energy** - For the brain and the body

- **Spare protein** - Necessary for other cellular processes and enzymes
- **Fiber** - Cleans out your septic tank

On the flip side are the poor carbohydrates. These are the ones that are usually man-made. These carbohydrates are low in fiber and other important nutrients and are absorbed quickly into the bloodstream, causing us to lose energy, feel hungry, and store fat quickly. Examples of poor carbs are bagels, breads, cakes, candies, cereals, chips, cookies, crackers, instant products (grits, oatmeal, rice, wheat), juice, sugar, and more. If these foods are consumed pre-workout, they will hinder the fat burning effect.

"If loving carbs is wrong, I don't want to be right."
~ Unknown

"Carb cycling" is one of the best ways to burn body fat.

Fact.

Our muscles and the liver are constantly full of stored energy, which makes it nearly impossible to burn fat. If glycogen is present, it is burned before fat. Excess carbs spill over into fat cells. The influx of low-carb diets do help in the reduction of body fat; however, trying to stay on a low carbohydrate diet all the time can be very taxing on the body and brain and is nearly impossible to maintain.

Carbohydrate cycling (consuming low carbohydrates for part of the week followed by moderate to even high carbs for the remainder of that week) can serve several powerful purposes:

- It is one of the fastest ways to drain carb stores, which will catalyze the use of body fat as the main source of fuel
- It shuts off the body's dependence on sugars and carbs as energy sources
- Lowers glucose and helps stabilize blood sugar to create aggressive body fat burning

I studied this method in 1995, and then I used it in 1996 to drop 22-pounds of body fat in 12-weeks for a natural bodybuilding contest. I still use it to this day for myself and numerous clients. It only takes a few days (three-to-six) to deplete the body's glycogen (carbs stored in muscles and liver). This allows you to eat good carbs the other day(s) of the week. Think of it as being in a body boot camp for half to two-thirds of the week and on vacation for the other one-third to one-half of the week. I prefer doing low carbs Monday morning through Thursday night and then increasing carbs from Friday morning through Sunday night.

Most people do best eating low carbs Monday through Friday and then increasing them on the weekend, Saturday and Sunday. Some people may prefer eating low carbs all meals with the exception of two meals per week, having a high carb meal every 72-hours. This way you can enjoy some of your favorite foods without feeling deprived. It typically takes three days (72-hours) to deplete glycogen. Those folks that need to lose more than twenty pounds will need to deplete carbs longer (five-to-six days) and replenish carbs shorter (one-to-two days).

I have seen numerous clients drop three-to-six pounds the first week, and some as much as 12-pounds. Most clients I have worked with in the last 27-years have lost between 20 and 40 pounds in 8-12 weeks using this type of system. Diets are short-term, but carb cycling can be done for a lifetime without even feeling like you are on a diet.

Tips for carb cycling:

- Try to eat every 3-4 hours until 2-3 hours before bed
- Eat 3-5 times daily (4-6 if training intensely)
- Weigh yourself only once per week
- Take weekly measurements and pictures
- Eat palm-sized amount of animal protein
- Women = 20-30 grams of protein per meal
- Men = 30-40 grams of protein per meal

- Eat mostly high fiber, low glycemic carbs
- No beets, carrots, corn, peas, or squash on low carb days (all too starchy)
- Avoid condiments like ketchup, BBQ sauce, and salad dressings that have lots of sugar (consider making your own to control sugar content)
- Most mustards, salsas, horse radishes, and mayos are fine, but check the label for sugar.
- No artificial sweeteners or non-dairy creamers (use stevia or monk fruit and real cream)

"Don't start a diet that has an expiration date…
Focus on a lifestyle that will last forever."
~ Unknown

A Don Story: Carbohydrate Indulgence

It was a hot and humid Saturday evening in June of 1996. My wife and I had just stepped outside one of the many back doors of a high school in Denver, Colorado. The only thought on our minds was eating. We had been training and dieting for 16 intense weeks for the Colorado Natural Bodybuilding Championships. Junk food had been excluded from our eating plan for the previous four months. My weight was down 22 pounds (192 to 170). Now we were done. Hallelujah! It was time to celebrate.

Jumping into the car, we raced to a local pizza and burger joint. Sitting on the car floor was a box of unopened Samoa's. These were the Girl Scout cookies we had been saving in our freezer the last couple of months for this very occasion. They would be our first treat for the celebration. Opening the box quickly, we split it down the middle, devouring the entire box of sugary goodness.

Sitting at the restaurant, our mouths watered as we scouted the menu. We relished the moment. Famished from weeks of deprivation, we each ordered and ate enough burgers, fries, pizza, onion rings, and desserts for four people.

After an hour or so of savoring every last bite, it was time to head back to where we were staying. It was a 30-minute drive, so we could partially digest our stuffed gullets. Ten minutes away from our destination, we spotted a supermarket. Looking at one another and smiling, we took the next exit.

Giddy, we chose the larger shopping cart over the smaller one. Up and down the aisles we sped. Frozen pizza, cereal, bread, juice, desserts and more, packed our cart. Reaching in my pocket I pulled out my wallet and credit card. The total was over $100! Unbelievably, this was about the same amount as our restaurant bill.

Arriving at our destination, we grabbed the four large paper grocery bags and headed in. It was after midnight, and we were exhausted. As tired as we were, the temptation of junk food beckoned, so we threw a couple frozen pizzas in the oven.

After sleeping for only about six hours, I was awakened by the sound of dishes in the kitchen. Looking in disbelief, my wife was sitting at the table eating her second bowl of cereal. How could she possibly still be hungry after the smorgasbord last night? I was typically the one to indulge. Joining her, I poured my own Jethro sized bowl of sugar coated goodness. After adding toast, jelly, juice, and pop tarts to the mix, we headed to a nearby water park for a Sunday of fun.

Glancing into a mirror, my body looked nothing like it had just hours before. The enormous amount of fast absorbing carbohydrates and sodium made my wife and I retain lots of water, giving us a bloated look and feel that would last for days. After our gluttonous indulgence, I was now ready to get back on a steady regimen of weekly carbohydrate cycling.

In order to keep your sanity and maintain a healthy weight for the rest of your life, I suggest eating low-carb for the majority of the week and then enjoying some high-carb foods on the weekend. Just don't go crazy like we did!

"Nothing tastes as good as being fit feels." ~ ***Unknown***

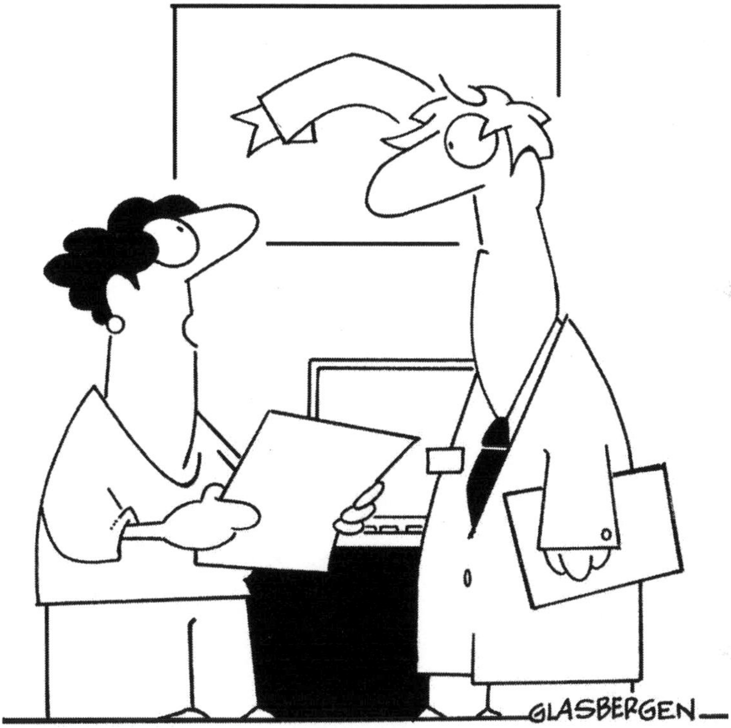

"Too bad it was a typo. I was doing pretty well on the low-crab diet!"

Sugar is responsible for increases in heart disease, cancer, diabetes, high blood pressure, obesity and the weakening of our immune system.

Fact.

The latest evidence reveals that the sugar industry suppressed studies linking the consumptions of sugar to heart disease and cancer. The group funding the study, The Sugar Research Foundation, cut the late 1960's project short and didn't publish the results. Nutritionists and scientists now warn that sugar, not fat, is primarily to blame for many problems in the modern American diet. It is a diet rich in *sugar* that has led to the epidemic in obesity, diabetes, heart disease, and more.

Doctors and researchers across the globe claim that the sugar industry may have intentionally kept the Sugar Research Foundation study from being published. Another study published in *PLOS Biology Journal* reports that the Sugar Association (former name of the Sugar Research Foundation) worked to suppress scientific findings on the harmful effects of table sugar nearly 50-years ago. Records show that the Sugar Research Foundation paid three Harvard Scientists in 1967 to make sugar seem less unhealthy and further, deflect blame onto fat as the main culprit in heart and other diseases. Doesn't this sound similar to what the tobacco industry did?

Decades of research show sugar to be associated with heart disease, diabetes, high cholesterol, kidney disease, and possibility cancer.

Nearly one third of common cancers, such as breast and colon cancers, contain insulin receptors that eventually signal the tumor to consume glucose. Lewis Cantley, a Harvard professor and head of the Beth Israel Deaconess Cancer Center, says some of those cancers have learned to adapt to an insulin-rich environment. "They have evolved the ability to hijack that flow of glucose that's going by in the bloodstream into the tumor itself."

In 1675, Western Europe experienced a sugar boom and diabetes increased, physician Thomas Willis noted. The early 1900s saw a huge increase in deaths from diabetes as sugar consumption continued to rise, according to Columbia University professor, Haven Emerson. In the 1960s, British nutrition expert, John Yudkin, discovered how increased sugar consumption elevate levels of fat and insulin in the blood, which increases the risk of heart disease and diabetes. These discoveries were all overshadowed by many other scientists blaming heart disease and obesity on saturated fat and cholesterol.

According to Richard Johnson, nephrologist at the University of Colorado Denver, one-third of adults in the world today have high blood pressure. In 1900, the number was a mere one in twenty people. Similarly, diabetes affected only one in 50,000 in 1900, while today that number is one in eight!

It turns out that sugar is the main culprit in these increased incidence rates, not fats, salts, or lack of exercise. The worst types of sugar are sucrose (table sugar) and high fructose corn syrup (HFCS). Both these sugars break down into triglycerides in the liver. Some of them stay, making the liver fatty and dysfunctional. Other sugars get into the bloodstream, causing an increase in blood pressure. With sugar cycling over and over again in the body with a poor diet, the tissue (muscle, fat and liver) becomes resistant to insulin. Now affecting one-third of American adults, metabolic syndrome (increased blood pressure, diabetes, and obesity) occurs. This leads to an increased risk of heart attack or stroke.

Sugary drinks are the worst. Check out the sugar in twelve fluid ounces of the following popular drinks: Snapple/40 grams; Monster/38 grams; Coke/39 grams; orange juice/28 grams; Gatorade/21 grams; Vitamin Water/19 grams.

"Two sodas a day appears to double the risk of dying from heart disease," says Jean Welsh, Ph.D., assistant professor of pediatrics at Emory University in Atlanta, Georgia.

Sugar hides in 74% of packaged foods, including most yogurt, cereal, bread, frozen pizza, cereal bars, sauces, soups, broths, salad dressings, and more.

The average American eats an astounding 22 teaspoons (⅕ pound) of this white poison every day! That's 77-pounds per year. At 4.2 grams per teaspoon and four calories per gram that's 370 empty calories per day and 135,000 calories per year. We should only be taking in a maximum of six-to-nine teaspoons (25-35 grams) per day. Nature made sugar hard to get; man made it easy.

Sugar is disguised by 50 plus different names: agave nectar, barbados sugar, barley malt, beet sugar, brown sugar, buttered syrup, cane juice crystals, cane sugar, caramel, carob syrup, castor sugar, confectioners' sugar, corn syrup, corn syrup solids, crystalline fructose, date sugar, demerara sugar, dextran, dextrose, diastase, diastatic malt, ethyl maltol, evaporated cane juice, florida crystals, fructose, fruit juice, fruit juice concentrate, galactose, glucose, glucose solids, golden sugar, golden syrup, grape sugar, high fructose corn syrup, icing sugar, invert sugar, lactose, maltodextrin, maltose, malt syrup, maple syrup, molasses, muscovado, organic raw sugar, raw sugar, refiners syrup, rice syrup, sorghum syrup, sucrose, sugar, treacle, turbinado sugar, and yellow sugar. How many of these are you familiar with? Be a vigilant label reader! Or better yet, buy whole foods made by the earth.

In 1973, 4.2 million Americans suffered from diabetes. The year 2014 saw a 500% increase from 1973 that reached 22 million!

In the movie, *Super Size Me,* researcher Morgan Spurlock gained 24-pounds of fat in one month from eating solely McDonald's food. His choices had hidden sugar that equaled about one pound per day. His blood pressure, cholesterol, and triglycerides all skyrocketed. His doctors were astonished and quickly advised him to halt the research. He persisted in his experiment, despite the doctor's dire warnings. The pounds he gained in one month, took Spurlock one year to lose.

We have become lazy because we have low energy; we have low energy because we eat too much sugar. Sugar is not just empty calories, it is toxic. "Sugar is poison by itself when consumed at high doses," said Doctor Robert Lustig, professor of pediatrics in the division of endocrinology at the University of California, San Francisco. "You could make dog poop taste good with enough sugar, and the food industry does."

Cereal was marketed in the 1800s as a convenient whole grain health food, but by the 1920s the food industry had transformed cereal into sugar coated and sugar infused flakes, puffs, and pops. Today, there are now an alarming 2,000 cereal products in the U.S. market, most containing high levels of sugar.

Sugar is just as addictive as cocaine or heroin! "Our findings clearly demonstrate that intense sweetness can surpass cocaine reward, even in drug-sensitized and addictive individuals," stated Professor Bernhard Baune, James Cook University, Australia, in 2007.

In addition to all of this, remember that sugar also makes us fat, tired, and hungry. The quick absorption causes insulin to be rushed into the bloodstream, and the excess gets stored as fat. Sugar also causes serotonin to be released. Converting to tryptophan, it makes us tired. Then, to make matters worse, sugar makes us hungrier still, by releasing a hormone called ghrelin. It is a vicious cycle, and people wonder what is wrong with them.

Receiving a Nobel Prize for his research on Vitamin C, Dr. Linus Pauling is known for being one of the greatest researchers in the field of microbiology. As part of this same research, he also discovered that eating any kind of sugar has the potential to reduce your body's defenses by 75% or more for four-to-six hours. Using this information can dramatically assist healing and prevent illness. It is especially important not to eat sugar when sick or healing.

"Sugar is eight times more addictive than cocaine.
And what's interesting is while cocaine and heroin
activate one spot for pleasure in the brain,
sugar lights up the brain like a pinball machine."
~ Doctor Mark Hyman, Medical Director at
Cleveland Clinic's Center for Functional Medicine

Raw honey has multiple health benefits that have been known about for thousands of years.

Fact.

Raw, unfiltered, and unpasteurized, this nectar from flowers is the only food on earth that doesn't spoil. Honey has been found in ancient Egyptian tombs dating back thousands of years. This golden delight is an alkaline-forming food that doesn't ferment in the stomach and can counteract acid indigestion. Containing 22 amino acids, 27 minerals, and 5,000 enzymes, this powerhouse of a food has been used as medicine since ancient times.

Eating honey helps with:

- **Weight management -** A University of Wyoming study shows that honey activates a hormone that suppresses the appetite.
- **Diabetes -** Honey reduces the risk of developing diabetes and helps aid medication used to treat it.
- **Sleep -** By restoring liver glycogen, the brain doesn't search for fuel, allowing you to go to sleep more easily and stay asleep longer. Eating honey releases melatonin by creating a small insulin spike and releases tryptophan in the brain. Tryptophan converts to serotonin and then melatonin. Melatonin helps the brain sleep naturally. (Remember that poor sleep leads to hypertension, obesity, type II diabetes, stroke, and arthritis.)

- **Counters pollen allergies -** Raw honey contains bee pollen which wards off infections by boosting our immune system and providing natural allergy relief. Local, raw honey is best because bees go from flower to flower in your area, which is the same offending local pollen. It desensitizes you to the fauna that triggers an allergic reaction. Some claim a tablespoon daily can act like an allergy shot, if you do it about one month prior to allergy season..
- **Provides easily absorbed energy -** University of Memphis Exercise and Sports Nutrition Laboratories, says raw honey is one of the best choices of carbohydrate for a pre- and post-workout. As a fuel, it is on par with glucose, which is used in most commercial energy gels. Honey was used by runners in the Olympic Games in Ancient Greece as a source of energy.
- **Wound/ulcer healer -** Honey-infused bandages aid healing. As a natural antibacterial, honey reacts with body fluids to make hydrogen peroxide, which kills the bacteria.
- **Natural cough syrup -** Honey has been shown to be as effective as over-the-counter (OTC) common cough syrups, decreasing mucus in just one dose. One-half to two-teaspoons at bedtime is recommended for anyone over the age of one year old as a natural cough suppressant. This is not touted because companies can't patent food or make enormous profits like they do from cold medications. I've used raw honey mixed in hot tea or hot lemon water as a cough remedy for many years.

Keep in mind, it takes 60,000 bees, collectively traveling up to 55,000 miles and visiting more than 2 million flowers, to gather enough nectar to make just one pound of honey. It is truly a precious resource.

"Eat honey, my child, it is good."
~ Proverbs 24:13

Blackstrap molasses is just another camouflaged sugar.

Myth.

Blackstrap molasses is the thick, dark syrup that remains after sugar is extracted from raw sugar cane. It is the byproduct of the sugar cane refining process. This bittersweet health food is one of the most hidden gems in the nutrition world.

The benefits of eating blackstrap molasses are:

- **Combats stress** - B vitamins, magnesium, and calcium all help combat anxiety and stress. Blackstrap molasses contains all of these nutrients.
- **Stabilizes blood sugar levels** - Blackstrap molasses has a low-to-moderate glycemic index of 55, which slows the metabolism of carbohydrates. It contains chromium, which increases glucose tolerance.
- **Relieves PMS symptoms** - Blackstrap molasses is high in iron. Women need more iron than men, because of iron loss during menses. Iron can improve mood and reduce PMS symptoms.
- **Helps prevent cancer** - High-antioxidant foods like blackstrap molasses help reduce free radicals in the body, which are thought to be a cause of cancer and other diseases.
- **Improves bone health** - It is a high source of calcium, promoting healthy and strong bones.

- **Lowers cholesterol and blood pressure -** Potassium-rich foods like blackstrap molasses help lower cholesterol, blood pressure, cleanse the liver, and support a healthy cardiovascular system.
- **Remedy for ADD and ADHD** - Blackstrap molasses has the iron and B vitamins that can help remedy ADHD naturally. These nutrients help support the nervous system and brain function, improving focus.
- **Treats arthritis** - It has anti-inflammatory properties that relieve swelling and joint pain.
- **Promotes healthy skin** - Blackstrap molasses contains lactic acid, which works as a natural acne treatment and heals other skin problems. Eating BSM also speeds up the healing time of cuts, wounds, and burns.

One tablespoon of blackstrap molasses contains:

- 730 mg potassium
- 115 mg calcium
- 15% daily value of iron
- 10% daily value of B6
- 8% daily value of magnesium

Molasses can cause digestive problems. If you have irritable bowel syndrome or experience discomfort, you may want to avoid this syrup.

"Your diet is a bank account.
Good food choices are good investments."
~ Bethenny Frankel, American television personality, author, and entrepreneur

A Don Story: Thick As Molasses

Awaiting the start of the annual Iron Horse Bicycle Classic, my client Les stood next to his metal steed. Laden with agonizing climbs over numerous mountain passes, this roughly fifty-mile course can test the most experienced riders. Having trained for months, Les was well prepared mentally and physically for this nationally recognized and legendary road race that stretches from Durango to Silverton, Colorado, on Highway 550.

Les wasn't your average middle-aged man. At 56 years old, he was a chiseled 170 pounds, standing 5'10" and was stronger than most men half his age. With the discipline akin to a soldier, his work ethic was second-to-none. On this day, he was quite possibly in the best shape of his life.

In addition to being Les's personal fitness trainer, I was also his nutritional advisor. For this event, I had designed a specific weight training regimen, as well as a nutritional plan for him that were both far from ordinary.

With its low glycemic index (slow absorption), very high potassium, and liquid form, blackstrap molasses was one of the secret weapons for his big day. Being such a nutritional powerhouse, it still amazes me that more athletes and average folks don't use this food product more often.

The race began, but I was neither a participant nor a spectator, as I was at home working on that gorgeous Memorial Day weekend. While mending an old fence in our pasture, I kept picturing Les on his ride. I imagined how his legs, as well as his heart and lungs, would be fairing on those long and steep climbs. Being from South Carolina, he wasn't used to training at high altitude. I wasn't sure if his gut would be able to handle some of the odd foods that I had him consuming prior to the race.

Still working on the fence at a fair distance from our house, my wife hollered something about Les. I was excited to hear the news. However, by the tone of her voice and the look on her face, I assumed it wasn't good. She said I needed to listen to the answering machine. I hesitated before pressing the play button.

His voice was clear and deep as usual, but there was something amiss. As I listened intently, he described different sections of the ride and how he felt both physically and emotionally. About halfway through (120-minutes or so) he said he started feeling nauseous. Abruptly pulling off the road and into a driveway, he said that he had to vomit profusely. He claimed the blackstrap molasses was the culprit. All of his hard work and now this! I was mortified and felt completely responsible. Unfortunately, there was still a bit more to listen to.

After tossing-his-cookies, so to speak, he gathered himself and continued the ride. With limited physical energy, but the heart of a lion, he battled onward and upward over another pass. Just beyond the summit, he said his bowels started speaking to him. He pulled over once again, but this time the expulsion was from the opposite end of his body. Soiling his bike shorts, he was now defeated. His wife had picked him up after only riding about two-thirds of the course. The blackstrap molasses was just not made for Les, I thought.

"What day is it, Don?" he asked towards the end of his message. "Does it feel like April first?" After pondering those questions for a few seconds while his voice fell silent, I realized what was happening. I had just been pranked! Wow, what a stellar job of fooling me he did.

Les completed the race in three-and-a-half hours, which was outstanding for his first bike race. According to Les, the blackstrap molasses had actually been one of the many factors that helped him achieve this goal.

"When your body is hungry, it wants nutrients, not calories."
~ Unknown

A gluten-free diet will make you lose weight.

Myth.

The vast majority of people don't even know what gluten actually is! There are many misconceptions surrounding this sticky protein that is found in wheat, rye, barley, spelt, and some oats.

First of all, many people believe that eating gluten-free is a weight-loss guarantee. However, most gluten substitutes are made from corn, potato, rice, etc. More often than not, substituting non-gluten carbs for gluten doesn't change the numbers on the scale, causing many people to become frustrated.

Just because something is gluten-free doesn't mean it's healthy, either. Like fat-free, sugar-free, and low calorie foods, gluten-free foods are typically not good for you. They are often loaded with sugar and have little to no fiber. The food industry spends millions of dollars marketing to make a product appear to be healthful and look delicious, otherwise you may not purchase that product.

Another fallacy is that *all* carbs must be eliminated when going gluten-free. Not true. Lots of different vegetables, fruits, and grains work well on a gluten-free diet. Buckwheat, quinoa, millet, amaranth, and teff are all examples of gluten-free grains. Some oats are gluten-free as well. If you choose a gluten-free diet, be aware that commercial products like sauces, salad dressings, meat substitutes, soups, breadcrumbs, chips, and more, often contain gluten.

Breadmaking changed back in the 1960s with faster production and cheaper goods. Called the "Chorleywood method" after the town in the United Kingdom where it was devised, modern bread making added preservatives, emulsifiers, and most significantly, enzymes to the mix. This method became the norm.

About this time, something started changing with our guts. Celiac disease, an autoimmune response to wheat and other gluten containing grains, has increased significantly since the introduction of manufactured bread. Irritable bowel syndrome (IBS) and inflammatory bowel diseases (IBDs) such as ulcerative colitis and Crohn's disease became a more common problem in the 1970s.

Many people started complaining about being gluten-sensitive or gluten-intolerant, termed non-celiac gluten sensitivity (NCGS). Some 29% of the U.S. population believe they can't eat the modern loaf of bread and claim to suffer from one or more of the symptoms, such as lightheadedness, aching joints, and upset stomach. My wife gets stiff joints after consuming gluten and my son gets headaches. We can always trace it back to gluten. Gluten has been found to cause inflammation in the gut, as well as inhibit the proper absorption of some nutrients in the small intestine.

The gluten movement has been supported by two best-selling books, David Perlmutter's *Grain Brain* (Little, Brown & Co, 2013) and William Davis' *Wheat Belly* (Rodale, 2011). Perlmutter, a neurologist, says gluten "represents one of the greatest and most under-recognized health threats to humanity." Davis, a cardiologist, blames gluten for everything from asthma, arthritis, multiple sclerosis (MS), and schizophrenia.

But research suggests that the problem may lie more in the enzymes that are added to these foods than the gluten. Alpha-amylase, which breaks down the starch in bread into sugars, may be the biggest culprit.

No one knows for sure what's going on, but something certainly is. The rate of celiac disease has quadrupled in the last 20-years, affecting around 1% of the population. However, Dr. Alessio Fasano, at the University of Maryland School of Medicine, states that the figure is much higher, around 7%. The real figure is much higher still, with only 24% of cases ever diagnosed, according to the Dr. Schar Institute in Italy, a premier resource for people with gluten related disorders.

The newest research shows that gluten peptides don't travel harmlessly through our digestive system. Instead, they pass through the gut walls and into the bloodstream, causing potential biological problems.

Researchers at the University of Milan found that the digestion of gluten resulted in exorphins (molecular fragments of wheat proteins), which have been found in the spinal fluid of people with autism and schizophrenia and thought to worsen the symptoms of these neurological diseases.

Gluten was also found to produce opioid-like effects on the brain, making one feel drowsy, one of the many symptoms mentioned by those who are gluten-intolerant.

There are many tasty (and some not so tasty) alternatives to the products containing gluten.

I recommend the following gluten-free products:

- Nature's Path Mesa Sunrise cereal
- Canyon Bakehouse 7-grain bread
- Blue Diamond Nut Thin crackers
- Bob's Red Mill all-purpose flour
- Pamela's pancake mix
- Mary's Gone crackers
- Tinkyada rice pasta
- Udi's pizza crust
- BFree tortillas

Another option to consider is sourdough bread. This old fashioned baking technique, thought to be used by Egyptians as early as 1500 BC, may help break down gluten in wheat.

A 2012 study published in the *European Journal of Nutrition* found that gluten-free sourdough bread may improve the healing process during the early stages of celiac disease. Because of its fermentation process, sourdough bread is rich in many vitamins and minerals. Most French restaurants and bakeries serve sourdough bread. Be aware that not all sourdough bread is made the same way.

Remember, most gluten-free foods have minimal protein, fat, and fiber and are therefore absorbed quickly. They are easy to overeat because they are inherently less satisfying than fat and protein.

"When diet is wrong, medicine is of no use. When diet is correct, medicine is of no need." ~ **Ancient Ayurvedic Proverb**

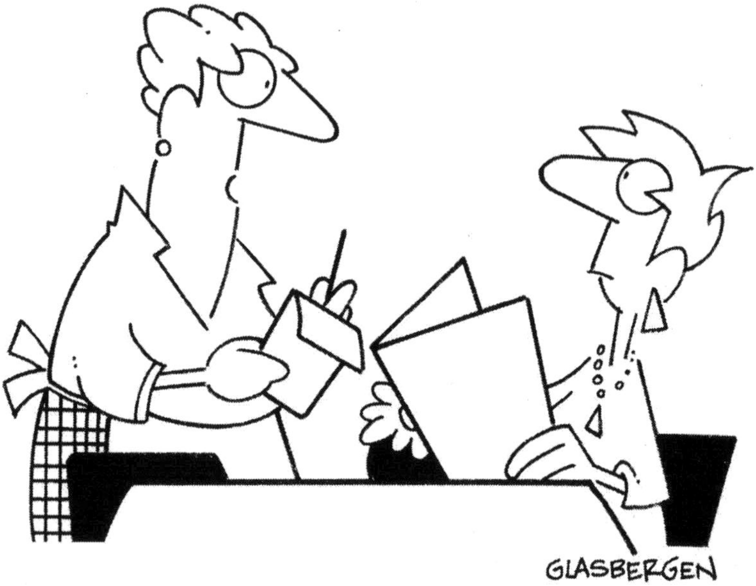

"If you're looking for something healthy, the menu is gluten free and printed with soy ink."

Fruit juice is not a healthy substitute for soda.

Fact.

With obesity affecting some 40-percent of adults and almost 20-percent of children, health care costs in the United States have skyrocketed to $170 billion per year. Sugar laden drinks are thought to be the main culprits of this obesity epidemic and increased healthcare spending. Soda and sports drinks are thought to be the largest single source of sugar in the American diet and contribute, on average, almost 150 added calories per day, which is why reducing sugary beverage consumption has been a significant focus of public health intervention. Most of the efforts have focused on soda, but not fruit juice.

For some reason, fruit juice has gotten a free pass. The average American adult drinks more than six-and-a-half gallons of juice per year. More than half of preschool age children (ages 2-5) drink an average of 10-ounces of fruit juice daily, more than twice the recommended amount by the American Academy of Pediatrics.

Parents are inclined to associate fruit juice with health, unaware of its relationship to weight gain and diabetes. They are hesitant to restrict it in their child's diet because fruit juice has been marketed for decades as a natural source of vitamins and minerals. For decades it has been sold in handy little juice boxes for packed-lunch convenience, specifically for children.

Despite all the government support and marketing, fruit juice contains limited nutrients, no fiber, and lots of sugar. A 12-ounce serving of orange juice contains the equivalent of 10-teaspoons of sugar, which is roughly what's in a can of Coke and other sodas. Though natural sugar may seem harmless, your body does little to distinguish between the sugars in fruit juice versus those in a soda or a piece of candy.

Drinking fruit juice and eating whole fruit are vastly different. While eating whole fruit like grapes and apples is associated with reducing the risk of diabetes, drinking fruit juice has the opposite effect. Fruit juice has more calories and concentrated sugar, and little to no fiber. Since fruit juice can be consumed quickly, it is more likely than whole fruit to increase carbohydrate intake. Research has found that adults who drank apple juice before a meal felt hungrier and ate more calories than those who started with a whole apple. Studies show that one-year-olds who drank fruit juice, drank more sugary beverages, including soda, in their school-age years. Excessive consumption of fruit juice by children has been linked to an increased risk of cavities, weight gain, shorter stature, increased blood pressure, and cholesterol.

We should encourage kids to consume water and whole fruits instead of juice. If we teach our children to eat healthier when they are young, they will most likely carry those habits for the rest of their lives.

Over the past decade, we have realized the harmful effects of sugary beverages like soda. Let's not fool ourselves into thinking that fruit juice is any different!

"Eat your fruits, don't drink them." ~ **Unknown**

Sports/energy drinks are healthy.

Myth.

The vast majority of the sports/energy drinks on the market are no better for you than soda. Sports drinks are not meant to be consumed regularly. They were originally designed to be used for athletes working at an extreme level of physical fitness for more than 90-minutes.

Taking a look at one of the most popular choices of sports drinks, Gatorade, for instance, the ingredients are water, sucrose, dextrose, citric acid, natural and artificial flavors, salt, sodium citrate, monopotassium phosphate, gum Arabic, glycerol ester of rosin, sucrose acetate isobutyrate, and artificial colors.

Three of the main ingredients in Gatorade are simply different types of sugar. While 12-ounces of Gatorade contains 21 grams of sugar (Coke = 35 grams), the regular (32-ounce) bottle of Gatorade that most kids and adults drink has 56-grams of sugar! With the ever increasing risks of childhood obesity and diabetes, sugar needs to be minimized.

The artificial food dyes (colors), such as Blue No. 1, Red No. 40 and Yellow No. 5, found in Gatorade, Powerade, and other sports drinks, are derived from petroleum and may increase the risk of hyperactivity in children. They have also been linked to cancer.

Gatorade is owned by PepsiCo, which dominates 75% of the sports drink market as of 2014. Powerade, which has basically the same unhealthy ingredients, is owned by Coca Cola and has roughly 20-percent of that same market.

Young athletes, parents, and the general public need to be aware of the adverse effects of these drinks. I have coached kids in baseball and basketball for the past several years. The parents and the kids are shocked when I state that I don't allow sugary beverages (only water) in our dugout or courtside before or during any practice or game. Unfortunately, I am an anomaly in coaching.

Water is the best option for children and adults who are engaged in low to moderate physical activity that lasts less than 90-minutes. Remember, our body is roughly 70% water.

For those kids and adults that are involved in high intensity activities lasting longer than 90-minutes, I recommend the following high potassium, low-to-no sugar, healthy electrolyte mixes:

- Ultima Electrolyte Powder
- Dr. Berg's Electrolyte Powder
- Optimal Electrolyte Powder
- Dr. Price's Electrolyte Powder
- Hammer HEED Electrolyte Powder
- Vega Sport Electrolyte Powder
- Diluted 100% juice with a pinch of sea salt

Stay away from the following sports drinks that are high in sugar, artificial sweeteners, artificial colors, and other harmful ingredients:

- Gatorade, Powerade, Powerade Zero, Pedialyte, Propel, Vitamin Water, ZipFizz, Lucozade Sport,

Accelerade, Cytomax, and any drink containing sodium benzoate.

Sodium benzoate is an ingredient in most of these drinks. When you combine sodium benzoate and acesulfame potassium (another common energy drink ingredient) you get benzene. Benzene has been shown to damage the cell's mitochondra, the powerhouse of the cell where you generate energy in the first place. Benzene has been found to cause cancer by disabling a cell's DNA.

Akin to a sports drink on steroids, energy drinks pose a possible bigger threat. With copious amounts of caffeine and other stimulants, these tonics can become addictive and may damage the heart and liver when intake is too high. As horrible as these are for adults, the side effects for kids are amplified.

The possible side effects of consuming too many "energy drinks" are:

- **Cardiac arrest** - in those with underlying heart conditions
- **Headaches** - from caffeine withdrawal
- **Increased anxiety** - in those with genetic variations in their adenosine receptors
- **Diabetes** - from excessive sugar
- **Insomnia** - from altering sleep cycles
- **Drug interaction** - ingredients may not mix well with prescription meds
- **Risky behavior** - some teens may be more likely to take dangerous risks on caffeine
- **Jitters and nervousness** - some may shake and be anxious

- **High blood pressure** - those with already elevated blood pressure could be at risk of stroke
- **Stress hormone release** - norepinephrine levels increase

The worst energy drinks on the market (in no particular order):

- Monster, Rockstar, Full Throttle, Red Bull, Burn, NOS, 5-Hour Energy, VPX Redline, Speed Stack, XS Energy, DynaPep, Spike Shooter, Bang

Monster has been involved in the death of five individuals, including a 14-year-old Maryland girl, Anais Fournier, who died of a heart attack after drinking two cans. Most, if not all of these concoctions have at least 160 mg of caffeine, tons of sugar or artificial sweeteners, and a list of other ingredients that are deplorable.

Supermarkets in the UK have banned sales of energy drinks to children under 16. Any drink with more than 150 mg per liter of caffeine must require proof of age before purchase. As of April 2018, South Carolina is looking to be the first U. S. state to ban the sale of energy drinks to minors. Let's hope other states follow.

If you're looking for an energy boost, you may just be dehydrated.

"Energy drinks like Red Bull may give you wings for a moment, but in time it takes away your basic physical and mental wellness and leads to disastrous psychiatric and physiological conditions."
~ Abhijit Naskar, neuroscientist and best-selling author

Artificial sweeteners are a safe alternative to natural sweeteners.

Myth.

Non-nutritive sweeteners, also known as artificial sweeteners, give us no sense of satisfaction and therefore make us overeat other foods. Eating an artificially sweetened fat-free donut will not squelch your hunger. Instead, you will be reaching for more food because nothing in the donut tells your brain that your hunger has been satisfied.

Research exposes many side effects to these addictive sugar substitutes that were first created back in the 1950s. They include:

- Cardiovascular disease
- Weight gain
- Headaches
- Migraines

Studies show that consuming artificial sweeteners increases your risk of metabolic syndrome (obesity, elevated blood pressure, elevated blood glucose, triglycerides, low HDL's) by 35% and Type II Diabetes by 67%.

These popular and dangerous artificial sweeteners have many names and are found in numerous processed and pre-packaged foods:

- Aspartame, Acesulfame Potassium, Alitame, Cyclamate, Dulcin, Equal, Glucin, Kaltame, Mogrosides, Neotame, Nutrasweet, Nutrinova,

> Saccharin, Splenda (600 x sweeter than sugar), Sorbitol, Sucralose, Twinsweet, Sweet 'n Low

They are also found in toothpaste, mouthwash, children's chewable vitamins, cough syrup, liquid medications, chewing gum, sodas, alcoholic beverages, salad dressing, frozen desserts, candies, baked goods, breakfast cereal, processed snack foods, prepared meats, diet juices, and other beverages. Carefully read labels to ensure you don't consume these dangerous, man-made chemicals!

A 25-year-long San Antonio Heart Study published in 2005, showed diet soft drinks increased the likelihood of serious weight gain much more than regular soda. The study found that participants who consumed one diet soda per day over seven-to-eight years were 65% more likely to become overweight and 41% more likely to become obese compared with participants who did not consume diet soda.

2008 research from the University of Texas Health Science Center (UTHSC) at San Antonio related a person's risk of obesity to their diet-soda intake. Compared with people who don't drink artificially sweetened beverages, those who drank more than three of these drinks per day were more than twice as likely to become obese in the next seven-to-eight years. This was verifiable even after accounting for the study participants' original BMI, age, race, exercise levels, and smoking and diabetes status. In 2016, UTHSC followed up and found that participants waistlines increased 3.16 inches among participants who drank one or more diet sodas per day; 1.83 inches among participants who drank some diet soda but less than 1 diet soda per day; 0.80 inches among those who didn't drink diet soda. Average waist circumference increased almost 400% more in the diet-soda drinkers than in those who abstained, over almost ten years.

An herbal sweetener gaining popularity is monk fruit, also known as luo han guo or Buddha fruit. This non-calorie natural sweetener is 150-200 times sweeter than sugar and has been used since the 13th century, when it was discovered by Chinese monks.

The potential health benefits of monk fruit include:

- Relieving allergies
- Cancer prevention
- Boosting immunity
- Promoting weight loss
- Improving heart health
- Helping control diabetes
- Providing anti-aging properties
- Providing anti-inflammatory properties

Add monk fruit to drinks like coffee, tea, lemonade, smoothies, soups, salad dressings, sauces, yogurt, oatmeal, or other hot cereals.

Stevia, another non-calorie herbal sweetener, is a choice for many foods. However, the taste can be an acquired one.

To naturally enhance the taste of foods, without adding sweetness, try cinnamon, cocoa, licorice, nutmeg, and vanilla. Lemon and lime juice (both very low in sugar) also work well for liquids.

"If man makes it, don't eat it."
~ Jack LaLanne, American fitness, exercise, and nutrition expert, and motivational speaker

Drinking water can increase energy, boost your metabolism, decrease constipation, and may reduce cancer.

Fact.

A human can go for more than three-weeks without food (Mahatma Gandhi survived 21 days of complete starvation), but water is different. One week seems to be the limit a person can survive without water, based on observations of people at the end of their lives, when water and food have stopped being administered. Three-to-four days would be more likely in a healthy person. Water is second to oxygen in the survival needs of the human body. Up to 70% of the body is made of water and every living cell depends upon it to function.

The rule of thumb has long been to drink eight eight-ounce glasses per day. However, should a 100-pound woman require the same 64-ounces as a 250-pound man? Even though this is sufficient for some, we all need different intake based on our size, environment, and activity levels. Drinking half of your bodyweight in ounces of water per day is a good rule of thumb. If you weigh 150-pounds, aim for 75-ounces per day.

Without adequate water, our brain function and energy levels drop. Studies show that mild dehydration (1-3% of body weight) caused by exercise or heat can negatively affect brain function. Mild dehydration can also have a negative effect on physical performance, reducing your stamina.

Can drinking more water increase metabolism and reduce appetite?

According to two studies, drinking 16-18 ounces of water can temporarily boost metabolism by up to 30%. Drinking 68-ounces in one day increases energy expenditure by almost 100 calories per day.

Drinking water half an hour before meals can reduce the number of calories consumed. One study showed that dieters who drank water before meals lost up to 44% more weight over 12-weeks compared to those that didn't.

Another study showed that people who drank at least five glasses of water a day were 41% less likely to die of a heart attack. As a bonus, drinking all that added water may reduce the risk of bladder cancer by 49%, colon cancer by 45%, possibly reduce the risk of breast cancer, and fill in your wrinkles!

Studies published in the *American College of Sports Medicine Journal* show that even mild dehydration can impair memory, mood, headache frequency, and brain performance. Dehydration develops from excessive fluid losses through urine, sweat, loose bowels, and inadequate fluid intake.

Dehydration is one of the most common causes of constipation. The food you eat travels from your stomach to the large intestine. If you are dehydrated, the large intestine soaks up water from your food waste, causing hard stools that are difficult to pass.

From a satiation standpoint, we feel thirst and hunger the same way. More in tune with their bodies, young children can more easily make a distinction between thirst and hunger. If you're feeling hungry, and you just ate a couple of hours before, try drinking some water instead of grabbing a snack.

Be mindful that beverages such as tea, coffee, soda, alcohol, and sugary drinks don't hydrate the body like pure water does. Caffeine laden ones actually increase the rate of dehydration. For an alternative to just plain water, try adding pure lemon or lime juice with a little stevia or monk fruit, if desired.

To remove toxins from your drinking water, stay safe by either purchasing a quality water filter or buying reverse osmosis water. Bottled water is not safer than tap water. In fact, there are fewer regulations on bottled water than municipal water systems.

Remember to add important minerals that were filtered-out back in to your water. A liquid variety of minerals from the local health food store or a pinch of sea salt will do the trick.

Try to drink 16-32 ounces of water first thing in the morning, before having that first cup of coffee or tea. The benefits are enormous!

"Drinking water is like washing out your insides.
The water will cleanse the system,
fill you up, decrease your caloric load,
and improve the function of all your tissues."
~ Dr. Kevin R. Stone, M.D., physician,
orthopedic surgeon, clinician, researcher

Yerba Mate may be the healthiest drink on the planet.

Fact.

Yerba mate is a South American beverage enjoyed six times more often than coffee in Argentina, Paraguay, Uruguay, and Southern Brazil, where it is "the national drink."

Containing an astounding 196 active compounds, versus 144 found in green tea, yerba mate has less caffeine than coffee and black tea, and gives you that non-jittery boost. One of six commonly used stimulants (the other five are coffee, cocoa, tea, guarana, kola nut), yerba mate triumphs as the most balanced, delivering both energy and nutrition.

In 1964, the Pasteur Institute in Paris concluded: "Containing practically all the vitamins necessary to sustain life, it is difficult to find a plant in any area of the world equal to mate in nutritional value."

Primary benefits of yerba mate are:

- **Promotes healthy weight loss -** Ursolic acid and oleanolic acid in yerba mate help to reduce body weight by oxidizing fat and increasing energy during exercise.
- **Enhances physical performance -** Yerba mate increases the reliance of fat for fuel during exercise. It may also reduce fatigue and improve muscle contractions.
- **Stimulates the immune system -** Saponins (phytochemicals) in yerba mate reduce the risk of certain cancers, improve bone health, and help

blood cholesterol. It is an anti-inflammatory that strengthens our body's defense mechanisms.

- **Incredible nutrient profile -** Yerba mate contains vitamins A, B Complex, C, and E, as well as calcium, magnesium, iron, selenium, potassium, carotene, phosphorus, zinc, chlorophyll, fatty acids, polyphenols, flavanols, inositol, tannins, trace minerals, antioxidants, and at least 15 amino acids. Mate tea also contains theobromine, the "happy" chemical found in chocolate.
- **Decreases cholesterol levels -** According to a study published in the *Journal of Agriculture and Food Chemistry,* yerba mate decreases LDL cholesterol and reduces the risk of various cardiovascular diseases.
- **Colon cancer cell killer -** Caffeine derivatives in mate tea induce death in human colon cancer cells and reduce important markers of inflammation, says Professor Elvira de Mejia, one of the leaders of an extensive study conducted by the University of Illinois.

I started drinking yerba mate in 2010 after reading about its many nutritional benefits, and I can attest to the clarity of mind and increased physical energy it provides (similar to coffee). I recommend mixing yerba mate with a little raw honey or a bag of mint or ginger tea to cut the bitterness of this beverage.

"Yerba mate gives you the strength of coffee,
the health benefits of tea,
and the euphoria of chocolate."
~ Unknown

A Don Story: Yerba Mate

Walking across a courtyard, I spotted Giancarlo, a student I knew at Fort Lewis College, who was headed my direction. He appeared to be smoking out of what looked to be a small bong or something peculiar. I assumed he was smoking marijuana. "No. It's mate," he explained. He was drinking mate the traditional way - South American style - out of a bombilla (gourd) with a metal straw. The steam from the hot liquid had given me the impression of smoke. In all the years I had been drinking yerba mate, I had never seen or heard of such a method. I was intrigued.

Giancarlo and his girlfriend had been members at my gym for a short period of time, but I had yet to get to really know them. We sat and talked at great length about his love of mate and his passion for making it a business. After traveling to Argentina a year earlier, Giancarlo became dedicated to bringing people together by drinking mate together. He would call his business "The Mate Exchange."

He and a friend from the business program would soon be entering the Hawk Tank Business Plan Competition, hosted by the Fort Lewis College School of Business Administration and Office of Alumni Engagement. It was similar to the TV show, Shark Tank. If they won, they would receive $5,000 seed money for their mate business launch. He invited me to attend the contest. I was honored.

With a stellar presentation of their business plan, the Mate Exchange won first prize in the contest! With 43 participants vying for the award, it was a big deal. They would be distributing mate throughout the region to local health food stores and more. I offered to let them sell fresh-made mate at my gym because I believed so much in its nutritional value. Giancarlo was very appreciative and excited for the opportunity to be in front of health conscious folks at a local fitness center.

After giving away samples and making a few sales, he and I ended up converting a small storage room at the entrance to my gym into a sales booth with a window counter. It was a convenient spot for patrons entering or exiting the facility.

For the next year or so, Giancarlo created and sold a multitude of fresh hot and cold varieties of mate blends at the gym. Offering mint, ginger, apple and cinnamon, cacao and habanero, and more, he tested and fine-tuned his concoctions with passion and precision. Members loved trying this unusual drink and conversing about its health benefits and origins.

Giancarlo's infectious smile, warm persona, and brilliant mind were extraordinary for such a young man. Men and women of all ages were drawn to this tall, dark, and handsome figure. His positive energy was contagious.

Tragically, Giancarlo passed in the spring of 2017. He was only 23-years-old. His smile, laugh, wit, and wisdom will forever be engraved in the hearts of those who knew him. I cherish the short amount of time that we had together and toast his spirit many mornings when I drink mate.

"It takes a minute to find a special person,
an hour to appreciate them,
and a day to love them,
but it takes an entire lifetime to forget them."
~ Unknown

Drinking coffee can potentially decrease the risk of numerous diseases and help you increase your metabolism.

Fact.

Recent studies from the University of Oslo in Norway show that whole coffee (as opposed to caffeine supplements) has potent anti-inflammatory, anti-aging, and chemo-protective properties. The vitamins, minerals, polyphenol antioxidants, and bioflavonoids in coffee all work together to help neutralize the harsher effects of the caffeine.

Studies show that coffee has the potential to decrease risks of numerous diseases: Parkinson's disease, multiple sclerosis, liver cancer, colon cancer, and type II diabetes. The healthiest coffee is an organic whole bean variety. Dark roasts - Italian and French roast, espresso, and Turkish coffee have less acid and less caffeine. With roughly 400 billion cups served every year, coffee is one of the world's most popular beverages. About half of all Americans start their day with a cup or two of coffee.

If consumed pre-exercise, coffee can have many functional benefits:

- **Increased fat burning -** Extensive research by Ori Hofmekler, author of *The Warrior Diet* and *Unlocking the Muscle Gene,* shows pre-workout coffee can increase your metabolic rate by up to 20%, increasing the fat burning effect. Chlorogenic acid, found in coffee, may also slow the absorption of carbohydrates.

- **Increased athletic performance -** Studies show an average of a 12% increase in athletic performance when coffee has been consumed.
- **Improved endurance** - Caffeine can reduce your perceived level of exertion by more than 5%, making exercise feel easier.
- **Muscle preservation** - Coffee triggers your brain to release a growth factor called brain-derived neurotrophic factor (BDNF). BDNF also works in your muscles where it supports the neuromotor, which is the most critical element in your muscle cells. The neuromotor is like the ignition in an engine. Degradation of the neuromotor is part of the process that relates to age-related muscle atrophy. Coffee may help maintain more youthful muscle tissue.
- **Improved micro-circulation** - Japanese researchers recently discovered that those who are not regular coffee drinkers had a 30% boost in capillary blood flow after drinking just five ounces of regular coffee, compared to decaf drinkers.
- **Pain reduction -** A University of Illinois study shows the caffeine in 2-3 cups of coffee, consumed one hour prior to a 30-minute workout, reduced the participants level of perceived muscle pain, possibly encouraging exercisers to push themselves a little harder. A similar study by the University of Georgia shows that drinking two cups of coffee an hour before training reduced post-workout muscle soreness by up to 48%.

Don't forget (ha ha), you can easily eliminate these health benefits if you add sugar, artificial sweeteners, or artificial creamers to your coffee. Caffeinated drinks like Red Bull, Monster, and others don't provide the same benefits as coffee, and in fact are harmful to your health as discussed before.

As is the case with most things, too much coffee (more than three cups per day) can have adverse effects. A University of Oklahoma study showed that excess coffee can increase anxiety symptoms, especially those with anxiety disorders.

Also, according to a University of Nevada School of Medicine's report in the *British Journal of Pharmacology*, a woman who plans on becoming pregnant should be cautious. Excessive caffeine from too much coffee consumption may reduce the chances of impregnation.

"Coffee is a drink that puts one to sleep when not drank."
~ Alphonse Allais, French writer and humorist

Chocolate should only be consumed on rare occasions.

Myth.

Chocolate is one of the most craved foods on Earth. Its origin dates back some 4,000 years to the pre-Aztec cultures of Mexico. Originally drunk as a bitter beverage, cacao beans were fermented, roasted, ground into a paste, and mixed with spices (chili peppers, vanilla, and a trace of honey) and water. Known as the "Food of the Gods" throughout history, chocolate was a symbol of luxury, wealth, and power. It was valued for its mood-enhancing and aphrodisiac properties. Unfortunately, in today's world, most chocolate on the market contains too much sugar. White chocolate, which is basically just pasteurized milk and sugar, has no cocoa. Look for chocolate that is high in cacao (at least 70%) and low in sugar.

Chocolate with a high cacao content is rich in antioxidants and is anti-inflammatory, helping to shield nerve cells from damage. Historic documents show that in the 17th Century Europe, chocolate was considered a potent medicine for treating angina and heart pain.

Recent science shows that resveratrol, found in chocolate (and wine), mimics the benefits of exercising and positively impacts the mitochondria by stimulating AMPK and PKC-1 alpha, which help to remove damaged cells and stimulate growth of healthy cells.

The Kuna people of Panama, known to consume up to 40-cups of cacao per week, have only a 10% risk of stroke, heart failure, cancer, and diabetes. A metabolic analysis from 2012 shows that chocolate can have a profound effect on health by decreasing cardiovascular disease by as much as 37% and dropping the risk of stroke by 29%.

Chocolate also has neuroprotective effects. In other words, it's good for the brain. The flavonols, natural compounds found in cocoa beans, can help us stay sharp with memory, problem solving, and other cognitive skills. Older folks will also benefit from eating chocolate, as it helps with attention, processing information, verbal fluency, and memory. Effects are even stronger in those whose brain functions have started to decline. Studies show that women, in particular, benefit after a poor night's sleep by eating chocolate.

Health benefits of chocolate:

- Anti-inflammatory
- Anti-carcinogenic
- Anti-thrombotic
- Anti-diabetic
- Anti-obesity
- Mental clarity
- Protects vision
- Neuroprotective
- Cardioprotective
- Improved liver function
- Reduced stress hormones
- Improved skin conditions
- Increased exercise endurance
- Improved gastrointestinal flora
- Slows progression of periodontitis

Remember to choose at least 70% cacao to minimize sugar and maximize the health benefits of chocolate. Options that are 85% cacao have only half as much sugar as the 70% cacao varieties. Look for bars that are high in cacao; low in sugar; have few additives and overall ingredients; no added flavor,; no added preservatives; not "Dutched" or processed with alkali; processed at a low temperature. I recommend the following varieties:

- Greens & Black (my favorite)
- Endangered Species
- Chocolove
- Alter Eco
- Pascha
- Pure 7
- Lily's
- Lindt
- Theo
- Taza

"Chocolate is nature's way of making up for Mondays."
~ Unknown

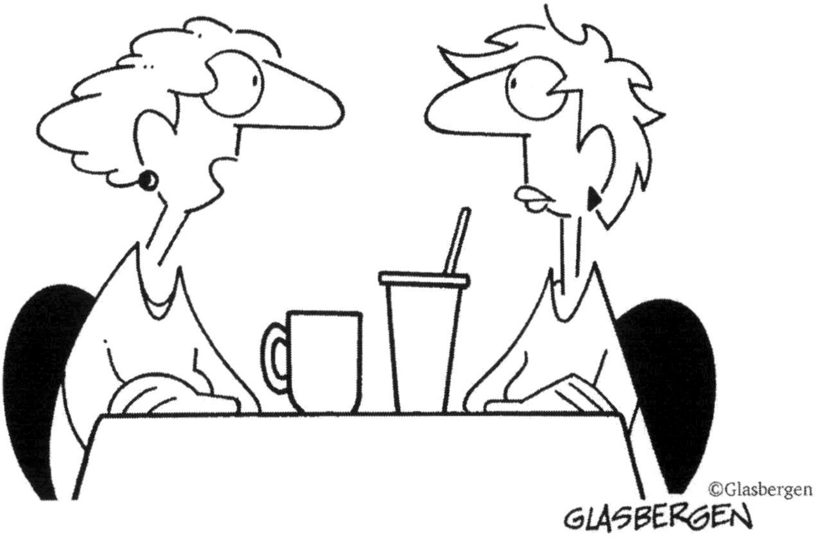

"I do weights for muscle health, cardio for heart health and chocolate for mental health."

Feed a cold, starve a fever.

Myth.

Traced back to a 1574 dictionary, this may be one of the oldest myths around. The belief assumed that eating food would help generate warmth during a cold and that avoiding food would help cool a fever. Recent medical science says the old saying is wrong. It should be "feed a cold, feed a fever." The body needs energy and eating healthy food, rich in nutrients is helpful for both ailments.

Drinking fluids when you have a fever is the most important treatment, as a fever dehydrates the body because of increased body temperature and sweating. Fluids for a cold are just as important. "You have to make yourself drink fluids even though all you want to do is collapse," says William Schaffner (not Captain Kirk), Chairman of the Department of Preventive Medicine at Vanderbilt University School of Medicine. Dehydration also causes more mucus in the throat and nose, clogging sinuses and respiratory tubes. Dry mucus makes it more difficult to cough. Runny mucus may be gross, but it is one of our natural defense mechanisms.

Don't force food if you're not hungry, but consuming liquids is vital. Minimize alcohol and caffeine since they tend to dehydrate. Taking a hot shower and eating soup is all good.

In at least two research studies, chicken soup (best made with chicken bone stock) appears to help fight colds. It thins mucus and clears nasal congestion so you can breathe better.

Research also shows chicken soup may have anti-inflammatory effects that can help ease cold symptoms.

Another great home remedy is hot tea. This also helps to thin mucus and hydrate the body. Low caffeine teas and yerba mate are filled with flavonoids, which are powerful antioxidants. Hot green tea with honey and lemon is one of my favorites when I'm sick. Over-the-counter remedies may or may not ease symptoms, but remember they certainly don't kill the bacteria or virus.

"Leave your drugs in the chemist's pot,
if you can heal the patient with food."
~ Hippocrates, Father of Medicine,
Greek physician

Kelp is a Supergreen.

Fact.

Kelp, along with dulse, nori, kombu, arame, wakame, hijiki, and agar, is a sea vegetable that grows in the nutrient dense coastal waters around the world. This superfood can grow up to one foot per day, reach 250 feet in length, and weigh as much as 30-pounds. Kelp has been a food staple in many Asian countries for centuries and is slowly gaining popularity in Western countries.

Kelp is considered a superfood because it is rich in vitamins, minerals, enzymes, amino acids, trace elements, and phytonutrients. Kelp contains calcium, iron, B vitamins, manganese, copper, zinc, and vitamin A. This sea vegetable also contains alginic acid, a unique compound that protects the body from absorbing heavy metals and radiation.

According to the National Institute of Health, kelp is known for having one of the highest natural sources of iodine. Iodine is essential for the growth and development of the brain. The *American Journal of Clinical Nutrition* states that iodine promotes better problem solving abilities and overall cognitive performance. Iodine is essential in thyroid hormone production, helping the nervous system and brain function.

Other health benefits of kelp include:

- Digestion
- Anti-aging
- Weight loss
- Antioxidant

- Stress relief
- Bone strength
- Virus protection
- Anti-inflammatory
- Blood clot reduction
- Decreased cholesterol
- Diabetes treatment and prevention

Kelp also contains fucoidan, a powerful cancer fighter that helps cancer cells die (apoptosis) in leukemia, colon, breast, and lung cancer. In addition, kelp contains fucoxanthin, which can help remove drug resistance in cancer patients undergoing chemotherapy treatments.

Kelp comes in many different forms; raw, powdered, cooked, and packaged, or as a supplement. I prefer the powdered version, which has minimal taste and like to add it to salads, eggs, and soups.

Warning: Ingesting large amounts of kelp can introduce excessive amounts of iodine into the body and overstimulate the thyroid gland, causing harm. There are significant health risks in consuming excessive iodine. It is important to eat kelp in moderation and it should be avoided by those with an overactive thyroid (hyperthyroidism). Try to eat organic kelp as to not get the arsenic, cadmium, and lead that is typically found in non-organic varieties.

"You can trace every sickness,
every disease, and every ailment
to a mineral (a nutrient) deficiency."
~ Dr. Linus Pauling, American chemist.
The only person in history awarded
two unshared Nobel Prizes.

Protein is an overrated nutrient that should be consumed minimally.

Myth.

"Protos," the Greek word for protein, means "first." This macronutrient should be considered number one in dietary importance, ahead of fat and carbohydrates. Protein is part of every cell, tissue, and organ. Dr. Spencer Nadolsky, a board certified family and bariatric (weight loss) physician, says, "Protein is King."

Proteins are the building blocks of muscles, tendons, skin, and organs. They are used to make hormones, enzymes, neurotransmitters, and molecules that serve important functions. Without protein, life would not be possible.

As important as protein is, there are many opinions on how much we need. Most nutrition organizations recommend a modest intake. The amount that the USDA (United States Department of Agriculture) recommends is used quite frequently. The DRI (Dietary Reference Intake) for the average sedentary man is 56 grams per day and for the average sedentary woman is 46 grams per day. These recommended portions may prevent deficiency, but it is far from sufficient for optimal health and body composition. Many factors determine the right amount: activity levels, physique goals, muscle mass, and age. Active individuals should consume .5 -.9 grams per pound of bodyweight (75-135 grams for a 150 pound person) per day, according to Nancy Rodriguez, PhD, professor of nutritional sciences at the University of Connecticut. The American College of

Sports Medicine recommends similar amounts for active individuals seeking to increase muscle mass.

Gaining and preserving muscle mass is not just important for athletes and bodybuilders. Growing children, as well as older adults who are at risk for age-related muscle loss, need more protein. In a study published by the *American Journal of Physiology-Endocrinology and Metabolism,* healthy adults ages 52 to 75 who consumed 1.5 grams of protein per kilogram of bodyweight, built and preserved more muscle than those who ate the recommended .8 gram minimum. "As we get older, our bodies become less efficient in using protein," Donald K. Layman, professor emeritus of food science and human nutrition at the University of Illinois says. "We need more protein to encourage the same muscle health." A lot of people out there think that eating too much protein is bad for the kidneys and bones, but those are myths, says Layman. "The only evidence that protein can be harmful to the kidneys is in people who already have kidney problems."

Animal protein provides all the amino acids (chain of molecules) in the proper ratio for us. Animal tissue is similar to our own. Choose hormone-free, grass-fed options when possible. For vegetarians and omnivores, quinoa, nuts and seeds, legumes, pea and rice protein, almond cheese, tempeh, and nutritional yeast are all good choices of protein.

Protein provides a multitude of functions for numerous body systems:

- **Muscle system** - Protein provides components that allow muscle contraction

- **Cardio system** - Protein maintains blood pressure and transports a variety of substances
- **Digestive system** - Protein serves as a digestion enzyme
- **Energy system** - Protein promotes oxygen based energy production inside the mitochondria
- **Detoxification system** - Protein processes potential toxins to be eliminated from the body
- **Endocrine system** - Protein serves as hormones
- **Nervous system** - Protein provides amino acids for neurotransmitters
- **Genetic system** - Protein aids in the formation of DNA and RNA
- **Connective tissue system** - Protein provides elasticity, fluid gel structures, and adhesiveness
- **Cellular system** - Protein provides structural integrity and protection
- **Signaling system** - Protein transfers chemical messages into and out of cells

"You are what you eat. Don't be fast, easy, cheap, or fake."
~ Unknown

Eggs labeled "cage-free" are a scam.

Fact.

Unfortunately, many people overlook the importance of what an animal is fed and how that relates to the nutritional benefits of that food.

Eggs are one example of this. The majority of the egg supply in the U.S. is from factory-farmed chickens that live in extremely cramped, unhealthy conditions. On these factory-farms, chickens are fed an unnatural diet of grains that severely affects the nutritional quality of those eggs. Unhealthy eggs, in turn, affect the health of the person consuming the eggs.

Regular (conventional) eggs from stores contain between 30 mg to 80 mg of omega-3 fatty acids per egg. However, hens allowed to roam freely in a pasture and fed a diverse option of greens, worms, insects, etc., can contain anywhere between 300 mg -700 mg of omega-3s per egg, as well as higher amount of vitamins, minerals, and antioxidants. This is the same thing that happens with grass-fed beef versus grain-fed beef.

Cage-free doesn't mean that the chickens actually go outside or have access to daylight. It only means that there is a small door somewhere that the hens could go outside if they were able to find that door in a giant coop with thousands of other hens. Caged hens can't forage, nest, perch, dust-bathe, or exercise - all of the things that they are meant to do!

Pasture-raised eggs are guaranteed to be the healthiest eggs available and the hens are treated the best. The next best eggs would be those from a local farmer who allows the hens outdoor space and feeds them a natural diet.

If neither of these options is available, a third option would be organic eggs or omega-3 eggs. These eggs would have at least been fed organic food and/or given supplemental flax or other omega-3 rich feed.

While pasture-raised eggs can cost between $5 and $7 per dozen, compared to $3 per dozen, keep in mind that is only 40-50 cents per egg. Eggs are one of the most nutrient dense foods on the planet. Isn't it worth 20-30 cents more per egg to upgrade your choice to pasture-raised? The taste alone should be worth the difference!

"Noise proves nothing.
Often a hen who has merely laid an egg,
cackles as if she laid an asteroid."
~ Mark Twain, American writer, humorist, entrepreneur, publisher, lecturer

The most powerful superfood is a plant.

Myth.

Plants like kale, chard, seaweed, and acai berries are incredibly nutritious. However, the most nutrient dense foods on earth are actually organ meats. Liver is arguably the most nutrient dense wonder food.

Benefits from eating liver or liver supplements include:

- **High in vitamin B12 -** Liver is good for our DNA, brain function, and energy.
- **High in vitamin A** - Liver is beneficial for eye health, bones, skin, teeth, reducing inflammation, staving off dementia and Alzheimer's disease.
- **Loaded with iron, selenium, zinc, copper, and chromium and more** - Liver contains many minerals that were once prevalent in our soil.
- **High in protein and low in calories** - Liver is beneficial for weight loss.
- **A good source of CoQ10 -** Liver is important for cardiovascular health.
- **Improves oxygen carrying capacity of blood cells**
- **Contains an unidentified anti-fatigue factor**

After a successful kill, our ancestors would eat the liver and other organ meats first. In fact, the liver was usually reserved for the "king" or leader of the tribe. Our ancient ancestors instinctively knew that the liver and other organs contained the richest sources of minerals, vitamins, and other nutrients. Wild animals are no different. They tend to go for the organ meats first as well, leaving the remainder of the animal for a later feast.

Liver can have a strong taste and slimy texture, and therefore doesn't appeal to many Americans. However, liver tablets and capsules are a great alternative as they have a mild taste and can be swallowed with a glass of water.

Jack LaLanne, considered by many as the Godfather of Fitness, was known for consuming as many 30 dessicated liver tablets per day and even more before a big event. Maybe this is one reason Jack was known for having amazing stamina while doing incredible feats of strength and endurance. Jack lived to be 96-years-old.

Vince Gironda, "The Iron Guru" and trainer of many famous movie stars from the 1960s, was also a big proponent of liver tablets. He recommended taking two liver tablets every waking hour during the day to prime the muscles with crucial nutrients. Vince believed that eating and drinking farm fresh fertile eggs, heavy cream, and liver tablets was better than taking steroids and certainly healthier.

While the quantity advocated by LaLanne and Gironda may be excessive, I would encourage you to add liver pills to your daily nutritional regime. Think of them as a food more than a supplement.

If you like the taste of liver, buy grass-fed meat without hormones, because liver can retain toxins from drugs and other chemicals.

"Liver is my number one most hated food. Oh, God I get sick talking about it." ~ **Guy Fieri, American restauranteur, author, television personality**

Testosterone is a hormone that is boosted naturally with food.

Fact.

Important for both men and women, testosterone is a hormone that helps build lean muscle tissue, increase feelings of well-being, increase libido, and sexual pleasure. Testosterone plays an important role in helping to balance estrogen production in women.

This hormone declines as we age, but there are natural methods of increasing it. Adequate sleep, proper exercise, reducing stress, and minimizing sugar and other fast absorbing carbohydrates are important for maximizing testosterone. The foods we chose can also play an important role in this process.

The best foods for increasing testosterone are ones that are rich in zinc and vitamin D3:

- **Tuna** - high in vitamin D. May boost testosterone by up to 90% according to a study at Graz Medical University, Austria.
- **Whey protein** - a Finnish study showed that consuming 15-grams of whey before and after resistance exercise, increased testosterone production by 25% and was maintained for 48-hours.
- **Olive oil** - consumed daily may increase testosterone levels by 17-19% over a three-week period.

- **Eggs** - the yolk's cholesterol is a precursor to testosterone.
- **Oysters** - high in zinc. Oysters help boost testosterone and are known for their libido-boosting effects. Other foods high in zinc include pumpkin seeds, wild-caught salmon, and sardines.
- **Coconut** - high in saturated fat. Saturated fats help produce most hormones, testosterone included.
- **Garlic** - contains allicin, a compound that lowers cortisol. With lower cortisol levels, the body can use testosterone more efficiently and effectively.
- **Cruciferous vegetables** - help to decrease estrogen in men, which help to maximize testosterone levels.
- **Grapes** - help sperm to be more active. Chinese researchers found the equivalent of 500 mg (5-10 grams) of grape skins raised T-levels and improve epididymal motility (sperm viability).
- **Cabbage** - full of a chemical called indole-3-carbinol, which rids men's blood of female hormones.

Symptoms of low testosterone include: low energy, fatigue, high blood pressure, decreased strength, low sex drive, loss of lean muscle, and increased body fat.

"I grew up with a lot of boys.
I probably have a lot of testosterone for a woman."
~ Cameron Diaz, American actor

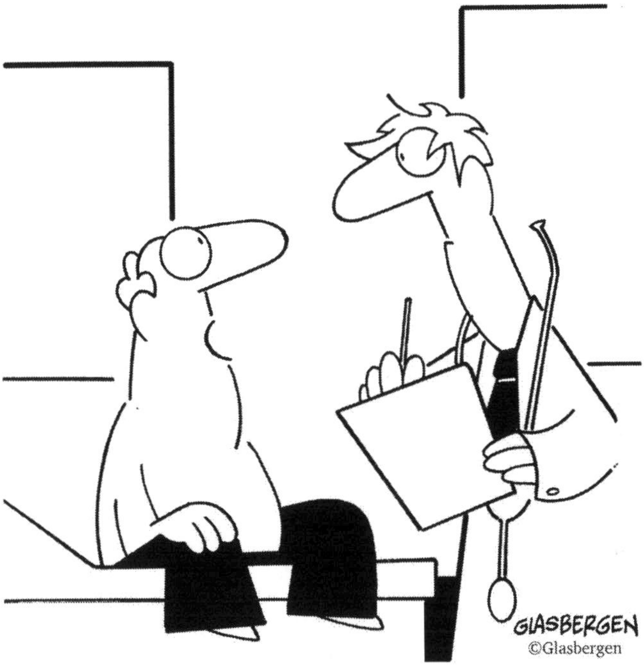

"You told me to eat more fish, but my weight stays the same no matter how many anchovies I put on my pizza!"

All salt is basically the same, causes high blood pressure and should be minimized.

Myth.

Regular table salt contains only two minerals, sodium and chloride. Sodium makes up 40% and chloride 60%. Other minerals are removed during processing.

However, unrefined sea salt is rich in 60-to-84 different trace minerals. These salt minerals are hard to obtain from the industrialized food that we eat today (because of a lack of nutrient-dense soil), but are still found abundantly in our oceans and seas.

The benefits of replacing table salt with unrefined sea salt include:

- **Helps avoid dehydration while balancing fluids -** Water follows salt. Too much sodium will cause water retention, while too little sodium causes dehydration and thirst.
- **Excellent electrolyte source -** Sodium, magnesium, calcium, and potassium are all essential to good health. These sea salt minerals are critical for a regular heartbeat, as well as muscle contractions.
- **Proper brain, muscle, and nerve system functions**
- **Digestive health aid -** Too little salt decreases the levels of hydrochloric acid (HCL) in the stomach, which leads to poor digestion.

- **Nutrient enhancer -** Sea salt helps maintain proper stomach acid, helping our bodies absorb vitamins and minerals. This is crucial for digesting and processing what we eat.

Sea salt can be both refined and unrefined. It is best to use the unrefined.

Himalayan Sea Salt and Celtic Sea Salt are popular choices. Himalayan salt (rock salt) is mined after being compressed for millennia or longer. Celtic Sea Salt, which is not mined, is higher in trace minerals and has a greater bioavailability (absorbs into human cells easier) than Himalayan Sea Salt.

Doctor Walter Kempner, a Duke University researcher from the 1940s, became famous for using salt restriction to treat people with high blood pressure (hypertension). Studies later confirmed that reducing salt could help reduce hypertension. However, scientific data shows there is no reason for people with normal blood pressure to restrict their sodium intake. If you already have high blood pressure, you may be "salt sensitive." Therefore, reducing the amount of salt you eat could be helpful.

Elevated blood pressure is a symptom not a cause. Salt reduction does nothing for heart disease because the cause of high blood pressure (and heart disease) is insulin resistance, obesity, and elevated triglycerides (Syndrome X) - not excess salt!

One of the best ways to minimize blood pressure is exercise and to eat foods high in potassium.

"Salt is born of the purest parents: the sun and the sea."
~ Pythagoras

A Don Story: Salty Joe

I believe it was Christmas, but it may have been Easter. The Roberts clan was gathered for a holiday feast. My mother's meals were highly coveted by all who were blessed to partake. With about 15 people sitting around the large dining room table, we were ready to indulge in the traditional event.

Sitting next to my brother-in-law, Joe, I was guaranteed to be entertained by one of his many colorful stories. Joe had been an athlete in school, a bull rider, shop teacher, high school football and basketball coach, and realtor. His stories were legendary, but on this fine day something else would be remembered.

Mashed potatoes, gravy, asparagus, dinner rolls, salad, and ham were the fare for the occasion. After salting my potatoes and asparagus, I passed the shaker to Joe. With my jaw dropped and eyes wide, I sat in amazement as he heavily salted his ham. He actually salted his ham! As you probably know, this is one of, if not the most, sodium laden foods on the planet. Everyone at the table was in total disbelief. Why would he want or need to salt something that is so salty to begin with? He just loves salt.

Joe recently had his blood pressure checked. His doctor was shocked. At nearly 70-years-old and having eaten massive quantities of salt for the past six decades or so, his blood pressure was low. The bottom line is Joe has never had high blood pressure, so large amounts of salt will probably never affect him like those that do have high blood pressure.

Whether adding it to eggs, chicken, beef, vegetables, or popcorn, salt has always been one of my favorite flavor enhancers.

Getting older, not being as active in sports, and actually using more salt on my food than when I was younger, I wondered if salt would ever affect my blood pressure. It never has. In fact, my blood pressure has always been low.

I know dozens of people who use copious amounts of salt and have never had a problem with high blood pressure.

"Give neither advice nor salt until you are asked for it."
~ English Proverb

Known as the gold standard, bananas are nature's best source of potassium.

Myth.

While bananas do have a decent amount of potassium (370 milligram/3.5 ounces), they don't even make the top 14 list.

Per 3.5 ounce serving, in milligrams:

- Blackstrap molasses 2,927
- Brewer's yeast 1,700
- Sunflower seeds 920
- Almonds 773
- Raisins 763
- Yams 700
- Dried prunes 694
- Peanuts 674
- Dried figs 640
- Avocado 604
- Quinoa 575
- Halibut 540
- Salmon 410
- Broccoli 382

Potassium is an electrolyte that helps maintain electrical and chemical processes in the body. Why is this third most abundant mineral in the body so important?

- Improves muscle tissue growth and bone health
- Stabilizes blood sugar levels and blood pressure
- Maintains optimal muscle and nerve function
- Keeps the brain functioning normal
- Maintains optimal fluid balance

- Builds stronger, fuller muscles
- Boosts the nervous system
- Prevents muscle cramps
- Keeps the body hydrated
- Improves digestion
- Prevents strokes
- Boosts energy

Potassium is required in somewhat large amounts to optimize the above benefits. The Institute of Medicine recommends 4,700 milligrams per day for men and women. Most people only get half of that at best. Potassium and sodium work in tandem, and we should eat a ratio of 5:1 potassium to sodium.

Those with kidney problems need to be careful not to overdo their potassium intake. Check with your doctor.

"Eating crappy food isn't a reward, it's a punishment."

~ Drew Carey, American actor, comedian, game show host

It's only slightly more expensive to eat healthy food than it is to eat junk food.

Fact.

According to the most comprehensive research of its kind, with 27 studies done in 10 countries, the *British Medical Journal* showed that it costs only about $550 more per year per person to eat healthy, whole foods (fish, vegetables, meat, fruit) than it does to eat unhealthy food (processed meats and processed grains, sodas, chips, etc.). That means that you only save about $1.50 per day eating junk food! (However, buying strictly organic or local will add additional expense.) The study doesn't include the enormous healthcare costs associated with a poor diet. Considering the national epidemic of heart disease, cancer, obesity, and diabetes, $550 more per year is a very small price to pay. In fact, you are likely to *save* far more than $550 per year in medical bills by eating a healthy diet. The added investment in good quality food will likely pay back in the first year and keep on giving for a lifetime.

Some people believe that a bag of chips is cheaper than a head of broccoli or that it's more affordable to feed a family of four at McDonald's, than it is to cook a healthy meal at home. They would be wrong. Neither is cheaper. In today's dollars, it costs about $24 to buy two Big Macs, one cheeseburger, 10 chicken McNuggets, two medium and two small fries, two medium and two small sodas. The cost of a whole chicken, plus vegetables, salad, and milk is about $14. It only costs $9 for rice, beans, bacon, peppers, and onion. (These are non-organic options and if you chose to buy organic, the cost would increase.) It may not be easy to organize your life to include shopping and cooking, but it's a choice! If you can drive to a fast food restaurant, then you can drive to your local market. Most people claim, "I'm too busy to cook." However, the average American watches more than five hours of T.V. a day.

As a society, we have become addicted to fast food and soda. The alternative to junk food isn't grass-fed beef and greens from trendy farmers (although both are great), it's anything but junk food: meat, fish, poultry, dairy, rice, beans, fresh vegetables, canned veggies, frozen veggies, peanut butter, and whole grains. The alternative to soda is water or unsweetened iced tea.

A 2009 Scripps Institute study shows that the engineering behind fast (hyper processed) food makes it addictive. The overconsumption of fast food causes neuro-addictive responses in the brain, making it harder to release dopamine. In other words, the more junk food we eat, the more we need to give us pleasure. This is the same thing that happens with drug addiction. We live in a food amusement park. With fast food on nearly every urban corner, it has become a cultural expectation. And, it is causing most families to not eat meals together anymore. It also causes obesity.

"Americans will eat garbage,
provided you sprinkle it with ketchup."
~ Henry James, American author

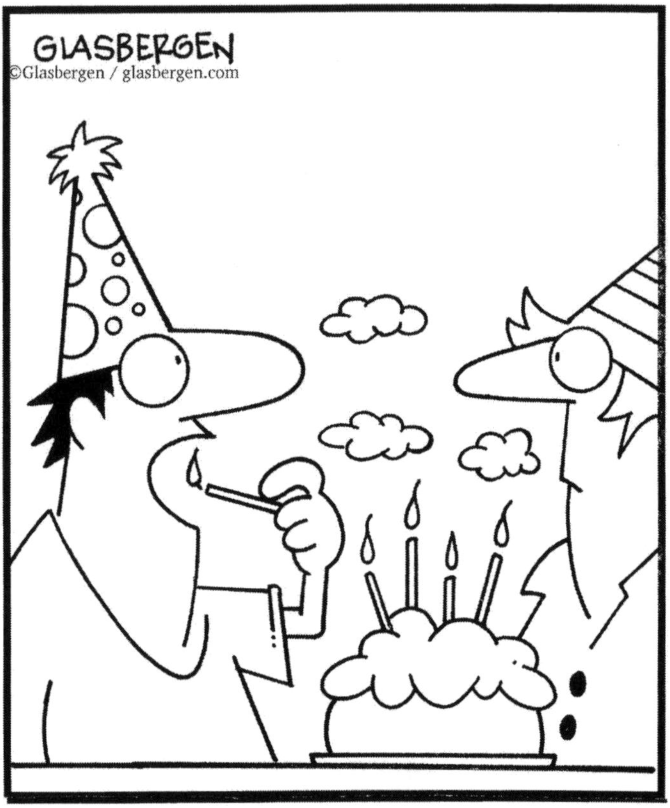

Diet Myth #173: Eating the candles on your birthday cake helps you burn calories.

Soy is one of the healthiest foods on earth.

Myth.

Because of brilliant marketing, millions of Americans believe that foods derived from soy are healthy. While fermented soy like tempeh, miso, and natto are healthy (containing beneficial probiotics), unfermented soy products like tofu, soy milk, soy cheese, soy burgers, etc. are not. Americans have been misled and manipulated into thinking unfermented soy products are good for them.

These unfermented soy foods contain trypsin inhibitors that inhibit proper protein ingestion and effect pancreatic function in many people. Unfermented soy also causes deficiencies in Vitamin D and B12.

More than any other legume or grain, soybeans contain a high concentration of phytic acid. This anti-nutrient binds to important minerals like magnesium, iron, calcium, and zinc and limits their absorption. The only way to reduce phytate content in soybeans is through fermentation.

Soybeans contain phytoestrogens which mimic the body's natural estrogen hormone. For women, this can cause an estrogen dominance, which can prevent ovulation, promote infertility, and stimulate the growth of cancer cells. Women with the highest levels of estrogen also had the lowest cognitive function. In men, high levels of phytoestrogens can lead to a testosterone imbalance, infertility, low sperm count, and increased risk of cancers.

Phytoestrogens are so strong that a baby consuming soy formula is consuming the equivalent of four birth control pills a day! In Japanese-Americans, regular tofu consumption in mid-life is associated with the occurrence of Alzheimer's disease in later life.

Thousands of studies link unfermented soy products to numerous health problems: Breast cancer, brain damage, hypothyroidism, cognitive impairment, immune disorders, food allergies, malnutrition, digestive problems, pregnancy problems, breastfeeding problems, reproduction, development disorders in infants, and more.

Contrary to popular belief, Asians only consume an average of 10 grams (two teaspoons) of soy per day, typically as a condiment (soy sauce or miso, for example) and not a main course.

The vast majority of soy produced on the planet is GMO (genetically modified organism). Ninety-percent of the soybeans grown in the United States are GMO. Soybean crops are also heavily sprayed with chemical herbicides, such as glyphosate, a known carcinogen.

Check labels to make sure the products you are choosing don't contain the following ingredients: soy protein isolate, soy lecithin, hydrolyzed vegetable protein, textured vegetable protein, or any other phrase containing the word "soy."

"You don't need a silver fork to eat good food."
~ Paul Prudhomme, American chef

A Don Story: Soy Products

My wife, Teri, moved to Durango, Colorado from Baltimore, Maryland in the summer of 1993. We met at Flexers Gym where I worked. She applied for a job, but we had none available. Fortunately, she joined the gym or we may have never met. We started dating only a couple months after she arrived.

Many things about her were intriguing, but the most intriguing was that she was a vegetarian. I didn't know any vegetarians. I naively assumed that vegetarians only ate vegetables. Little did I know that they also eat eggs and even dairy if they are lacto-ovo vegetarians. True vegans, like her brother, Jimmy, don't eat eggs or dairy. Jimmy, and their sister Lori, were instrumental in Teri's switch from an omnivore diet to a vegetarian one.

Teri's daily food regimen included a variety of vegetables and fruits, as well as numerous soy products: soy milk, tofu, tempeh, soy burgers, soy protein bars, and more. I, on the other hand, was and still am a carnivore; well, at least an omnivore. I eat lots of vegetables, nuts, seeds, whole grains, and fruit, but various meats and fish satisfy me like no other foods do. I wasn't accustomed to these somewhat bland and boring meat substitutes that were her staple. I tried most of her soy foods and would eat them on occasion, especially if no other options were available. I assumed they were healthy since they came from soybeans.

Teri continued on this vegetarian quest for a few more years until she became allergic to soy. The first sign was acne. She started developing pimples on her face. Even in her twenties, she looked like a teenager again.

Researching allergens, we realized that soy is one of the top allergens. What we didn't realize until many years later is that soy has a dark side. We now know that we were duped into believing that most soy, with the exception of fermented soy, is really not a health food at all and is not recommended.

Although vegetables are a top priority, Teri is no longer a vegetarian. Instead, she eats a wide variety of foods from all food groups.

"Learn how to cook.
Try new recipes.
Learn from your mistakes.
Be fearless.
And above all-have fun!"
~ Julia Child, American chef

More than ninety percent of cancer is the result of a poor diet and an unhealthy lifestyle.

Fact.

The lifetime risk of developing cancer is approximately 38.4% based on 2013-2015 data. In 2015, there were an estimated 15,112,098 people living with cancer of any kind in the United States.

The latest research shows that only five-to-ten percent of cancer cases are caused by damaged DNA. The rest is caused by poor food choices, lack of exercise, exposure to toxins, stress, and more. Surging by 300% since the 1970s, this second leading cause of death in the United States is expected to surpass heart disease by 2020.

From the early 1980s to the early 1990s, childhood cancer, which is the second leading cause of death in children after accidents, has increased by 37-percent.

Cancer is not a genetic disorder, but rather a metabolic disorder. Conventional treatments of radiation, chemotherapy, and surgery are still the norm, despite the studies that show more than 90% of cancer is directly related to diet and lifestyle.

Not a single disease, cancer amounts to over 100 different diseases. With no two people having the same immune system, toxin build up, microbiome (gut health) or metabolism, cancer is highly individualized and therefore can be difficult to treat.

According to 1931 Nobel Prize winner, Otto Warburg, when the mitochondria in a cell fail, that cell will become cancerous. Many things can cause cancer: Genetic mutations, radiation, toxins, bacteria, viruses, stress, and more.

Our bodies operate on water, food, and energy. Aside from getting the proper amount of rest, exercising, and drinking enough good quality water, what we eat has a lot to do with detoxing.

"If doctors were to study nutrition in greater depth, they would find that we are indeed what we eat because the cells of our food get broken down and transferred into the cells of our body... What we eat and drink directly affects our vessels and tissues, making them more or less inflamed depending on what we put into our bodies," wrote Dr. Kelly Turner, PhD, author of New York Times bestseller *Radical Remission.*

With more than 80,000 hazardous chemicals polluting the air we breathe, food we eat, water we drink, skin care we use, and cleaning products we employ, it's no wonder we are toxic. Scientists speculate that the average person carries more than 700 known toxins in their blood, skin, liver, brain tissue, fat tissue, digestive tract, and other parts of their bodies.

The following lists of foods and herbs are used for detoxing, gut health, and fighting inflammation and are provided by Dr. Nasha Winters, ND and Jess Higgins Kelly, MNT, best-selling co-authors of *The Metabolic Approach to Cancer*. Dr. Nasha Winters was selected by the Medical and Scientific Committee Chairs to be a keynote speaker at the International Medical Meeting in Germany in 2018. Winters was also the keynote speaker on alternative therapies for cancer in 2016 at Johns Hopkins University. She is a two-time survivor of stage IV ovarian cancer.

The most beneficial detox foods for cancer are:

- **Whey protein powder** (organic, pastured, unsweetened) - helps produce glutathione, a powerful antioxidant
- **Eggs** (from pastured chickens) - are rich in sulfur, which eliminates heavy metals, regenerates, repairs and rebuilds all the cells in the body
- **Lemons** - prevents carcinogenesis (initiation of cancer formation) and helps remove heavy metals
- **Wild Alaskan salmon** - high in B12 and selenium, which help form glutathione, a powerful antioxidant
- **Artichokes** - a low carb vegetable that help regenerate and protect the liver
- **Broccoli** - another low carb vegetable that helps remove pollutants, along with brussels sprouts and cauliflower
- **Beets and beet greens** - enhance the immune function
- **Chlorophyll** (green pigment in algae and plants) - accelerates the excretion of several environmental carcinogens
- **Chlorella** (green algae)- absorbs heavy metals
- **Dandelion greens and roots** - good as a liver tonic and also promotes microbiome health

- **Milk thistle** - a potent antioxidant that is powerful medicine for the liver, but poisonous to touch

Greek physician, Hippocrates, the "Father of Medicine," said, "All disease begins in our gut." What happens in our intestines (gut) is vital for our health. Our gut health (microbiome) makes up roughly 70-80 percent of our immune system. You can think of your immune system as fundamentally situated in our digestive tract.

The best foods for supporting our gut health:

- **Black raspberries** - a high fiber, low sugar fruit, containing ellagic acid, a potent antibacterial, antiviral, and anti-carcinogen
- **Sauerkraut, kimchi, and miso** - provide billions of naturally occurring probiotics for our gut health
- **Leeks -** a low carb vegetable that is high fiber, vitamin K, and has anticancer properties
- **Radishes** - an easy to grow and low glycemic root vegetable; a great source of arabinogalactan, a unique dietary fiber that attacks cancer cells and inhibits metastasis and protects against radiation damage
- **Wild asparagus** - low carb vegetable, rich in saponins, a phytonutrient that is a natural antibiotic
- **Umeboshi (Japanese salt plums) and Umeboshi Vinegar** - a fermented and alkalizing food aid used for digestion and nutrient absorption

Foods, herbs, and supplements that minimize inflammation are:

- **Turmeric** - used in Ayurvedic medicine for centuries, turmeric contains curcumin that has an unprecedented amount of anticancer benefits and is considered a "multifunctional" drug because it can regulate the activity of several targets involved with carcinogenesis
- **Green apples, onions, and capers** - all contain quercetin, the most powerful flavonoid known to man; quercetin is a free radical scavenger and anti-inflammatory
- **Boswellia -** plant that produces frankincense, an anti-inflammatory
- **Ginger** - is a powerful anti-inflammatory, and is used as a stomach settler and nausea reducer
- **Walnuts, chia seeds, wild salmon, herring, mackerel, sardines, cold pressed extra virgin olive oil, dark green leafy vegetables -** all high in Omega-3 fatty acids, which are anti-inflammatory.
- **Kale, spinach, and wild grasses** - all high in alpha-linolenic acid, the building block of Omega-3 fatty acids
- **Fennel** - contains powerful phytonutrients and is highly anti-inflammatory; also used as a digestive aid
- **Dark chocolate and cocoa powder -** have more polyphenols and contain higher levels of antioxidants than green tea, and both are high in magnesium; choose 80% or higher cacao for the greatest benefits with the lowest sugar content

- **Organic red wine** - contains resveratrol, a unique antioxidant that increases glutathione, minimizes oxidation, and acts as a phytoestrogen; red wine is full of tannins, which also show an anticancer effect (resveratrol supplements don't have the same effects)

Foods that block new cancers and cancer growth are:

- **Cherry tomatoes -** inhibit cell growth
- **Parsley, celery, chamomile tea** - all contain apigenin, a plant flavonoid that fights breast, ovarian, and colon cancers
- **Chaga mushroom** - a powerful antioxidant and is used to decrease blood sugar, as well as stimulate the immune system; paired with wild oregano, it has better absorption in the body; in cultures where people consume it daily, they have found little to no cancer
- **Chili peppers** - a chemo alternative and tumor suppressor; frequent consumption of spicy foods drops your risk of dying from cancer by 14%, most likely due to the anti-inflammatory effects
- **Cartilage** - found in collagen-rich bones from beef, chicken, and fish
- **Aloe juice** - a plant of immortality, it has been traced back 6,000 years to Egypt; aloe is a powerful antioxidant with medicinal uses, like repairing or preventing gastric inflammation
- **Green tea** - rich in catechins (flavonoids) and is a well-known and widely accepted anticancer beverage
- **Ginseng** - comes in three varieties - American, Siberian and panax; restores energy and is a rich

source of polysaccharides, flavonoids, ginsenosides, volatile oils, amino acids, and vitamins

Unfortunately, cancer has been prevalent in my family for generations.

Having lost my father, aunts, uncles, grandfather, friends, and clients all at early ages due to various forms of cancer, this is a very important topic to me.

Knowing that a healthy lifestyle is the most important factor in preventing cancer has motivated me for decades to teach my clients to eat right and exercise regularly, and to follow my own advice.

"He who has health, has hope.
And he who has hope, has everything."
~ Thomas Carlyle, philosopher

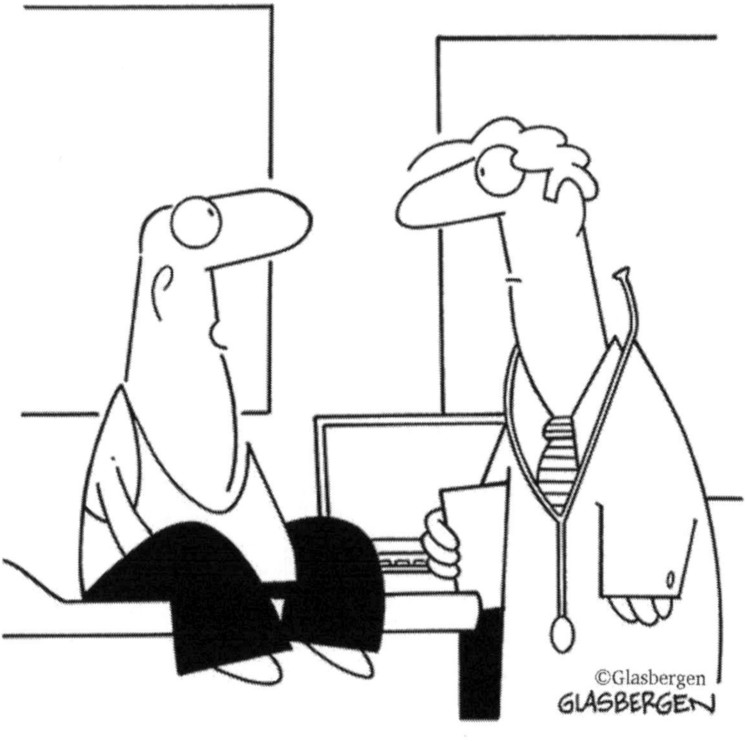

"You told me to eat 5 fruits and vegetables every day. Today I had 3 raisins and 2 peas."

Fresh fruits and vegetables are always more nutritious than frozen varieties.

Myth.

As you know, fruits and vegetables are among the most nutritious and delicious foods on the planet.

While fresh produce is normally the preferred choice, sometimes frozen is actually healthier. In several instances, the fruits and vegetables you purchase at the grocery store aren't at their nutritional peak. On the other hand, frozen produce is picked when ripe and then frozen, locking in the nutrition. Frozen fruits and vegetables actually have more nutrients than fresh produce when not in season. Produce picked too early may lose as much as 50% of its nutritional value.

In the U.S., fruits and vegetables may spend several weeks in transit before arriving at their destination.

Overall, fruits and vegetables from the garden or local farmers market are healthier than frozen ones. Be mindful to select frozen produce that doesn't have added salt. Also, when cooking, lightly steam, bake, or sauté vegetables instead of overcooking them.

Even though my family eats a lot of fresh vegetables, especially in the summertime, we have frozen vegetables often. Some of our favorites include a fajita mix of frozen bell peppers and onions, which are great in egg dishes or as a side dish with meats. Also, the broccoli and cauliflower combination goes well with many dishes. If trying to lose weight, be careful not to overindulge in the corn and peas, as they are starchy and may delay your progress.

One of my favorite ways to prepare a smoothie is to use frozen berries, which are low in sugar, combined with half of a banana, protein powder, and water or unsweetened almond or coconut milk. This combination is delicious, nutritious, economical, and easy.

"Knowledge is knowing a tomato is a fruit.
Wisdom is not putting it in a fruit salad."
~ Miles Kington, British journalist

Organic food is healthier than conventional food.

Fact.

While some studies show that organic food is not more nutritious than conventional food, other studies show just the opposite. However, nutritional content shouldn't be the most important factor to consider for one's health. Pesticide content should be a primary concern.

Even though pesticides are legal, that doesn't mean they are safe. While the 1996 Quality Protection Act helped to minimize the number and quantity of harmful pesticides used, the EPA uses a safety standard of "reasonable certainty of no harm." When uncertainty is combined with minimal long-range studies on the harm of pesticides, the effects of these chemicals are unknown.

Pesticides are poisons designed to kill bugs, weeds, animals, and more. Would you rather eat a poison or not eat a poison? Consuming a substance designed to kill life when other options are available is an interesting decision. Why make that choice?

DDT (dichlorodiphenyltrichloroethane), for instance, an organic insecticide (pesticide specifically targeted to kill insects) that everyone thought was safe, was in fact very dangerous and was banned in 1972. The effects of DDT were so powerful that it's still showing up in the bodies of people today, including those born after DDT was banned. Long lasting pesticides are still found in nature, in our water systems and soil.

In addition, runoff from pesticides used on farms is known to kill plants, trees, animals, and cause pollution. Pesticides are absorbed by the body and remain there long after you ingest them, building up as time goes by. Pesticides potentially cause health problems in people as well. They are believed to induce devastating and life-long diseases (from respiratory problems to cancer), and deformities in fetuses and children.

Symptoms of exposure (ingestion, inhalation, or skin contact) to pesticides:

- Eye and skin irritation
- Nausea, vomiting, diarrhea
- Headache, loss of consciousness
- Extreme weakness, seizures and/or death
- Respiratory tract irritation, sore throat and/or cough

Glyphosate, one of the world's most widely used herbicides (a type of pesticide) in current agriculture, has been the subject of scientific controversy for a number of years, especially since the introduction of glyphosate-tolerant genetically modified crops, like certain types of corn and soybean. Glyphosate can affect human erythrocytes in vitro, disrupt endocrine activity, and promote carcinogenicity in mice. In addition, glyphosate has been shown to cause major disruption to human gut bacteria.

Glyphosate-based herbicides, like the popular "Roundup," can act as an endocrine disruptor and cause DNA damage in humans as well as promote cell death in the testicular cells of animals. Many believe that there is a correlation between glyphosate and health deterioration in the U.S.

In 2013, researchers from MIT (Massachusetts Institute of Technology) concluded that glyphosate is likely to contribute to the development of autism, Alzheimer's disease, cancer, depression, infertility, inflammatory bowel diseases, liver disease, and Parkinson's disease.

The World Health Organization has classified glyphosate as a probable human carcinogen and a mitochondrial toxin. In 2018, a jury awarded $289 million to a groundskeeper who contracted non-Hodgkin's lymphoma after using Roundup. There are 4,000 more cases against Monsanto (creator of Roundup) that will be starting soon.

Many people believe that organic food is just too expensive. While this can certainly be the case, conventional foods have hidden costs, such as healthcare costs and costs associated with cleaning up the environment after pesticides and other chemicals wreak havoc on the land.

Be aware that other labels, such as locally grown, natural, and free-range do not mean the same thing as organic. Products labeled with the USDA Organic Seal must be grown and processed under strict rules and regulations. These other labels don't have the same requirements.

Many people believe that organic farming is far too expensive and is therefore not capable of feeding the world. However, long-term studies from Iowa State University found that organic growing methods produce similar yields to conventional methods, with the added benefit that organic methods result in better soil quality. In addition, longitudinal studies called "The Farming Systems" Trial, a 35-year-long project, conducted by the Rodale Institute, demonstrates that organics can feed the world while providing environmental benefits that conventional foods cannot.

Unfortunately, organic doesn't always mean pesticide-free. Residue from pesticides may be present in the soil, blown in by the wind, or carried in water runoff from neighboring crops. When in doubt, buy food locally, seasonally, and transparently grown to minimize exposure to these toxins.

"Every major food company now has an organic division. There's more capital going into organic agriculture than ever before."

~ Michael Pollan, Harvard professor, UC Berkeley professor, American author, and journalist

Apple cider vinegar is a wonder food that can help with a number of ailments.

Fact.

The healing powers of vinegar have been traced back thousands of years, to about 3,000 BC. Apple cider vinegar has been used to prevent and cure a number of ailments: arthritis, acid reflux, high blood pressure, constipation, and heartburn just to name a few. Hippocrates, a Greek physician used it to treat his patients between 460-370 BC. Containing acetic acid, a natural bacteria fighter, it was even used as an antiseptic during the Civil War.

Organic apples, one of the most nutritious foods available, contain over 40 vitamins, minerals, enzymes, and amino acids. Apple cider vinegar, with only three calories per tablespoon, detoxifies and purifies various organs in the body.

The most popular vinegar in the natural health community, apple cider vinegar is a natural disinfectant and food preservative. It breaks down fatty mucus and phlegm deposits within the body, improving the health and functions of organs such as the kidneys, bladder, and liver.

Its most successful application is stabilizing blood sugar. Apple cider vinegar has been shown to decrease blood glucose by as much as 34%, according to a 2009 Japanese study. High blood sugar is believed to be the major cause of aging.

Apple cider vinegar contains chlorogenic acid, shown to protect LDL particles from being oxidized. A 2004 Japanese study showed that apple cider vinegar may also kill cancer cells and possibly shrink tumors. It flushes out harmful toxins from the body and assists in weight control. Another study showed that daily intake of apple cider vinegar led to reduced body fat, smaller waist circumference, decreased blood triglycerides, and weight loss. It oxidizes the blood. Diseases don't do well in an oxygen-rich environment.

Apple cider vinegar also reduces the risk of high blood pressure and minimizes toxic substances and harmful bacteria. It can also promote healthy digestion, assimilation, and elimination.

It is strong tasting, so it is best mixed with water, and if necessary, add a little raw honey. I prefer about two tablespoons of this vinegar mixed in 16-ounces of water with added lemon or lime juice (1-2 ounces). Buy only raw apple cider vinegar to get all the enzymatic properties. It works best when adequate water is ingested to help carry out the toxins we ingest or are exposed to everyday. My favorite brand is Braggs Apple Cider Vinegar.

"Live modern, train old, eat ancient."

~ Unknown

Bone broth is an overrated, so called health food, that is basically just soup.

Myth.

The term "bone broth" is a bit of a misnomer. Broths are typically made from meat, while stocks are made from bones, thus "bone broth" could be considered an oxymoron. This magic elixir now commonly sold as "bone broth" is made from the bones of animals. It is said by some cultures in South America to have mystical powers and is taking America by storm. The paleo movement may have something to do with its present-day popularity.

Our hunter ancestors started making bone broth out of necessity. Tossing out animal parts was inconceivable. Every part of the animal was used, not just the flesh that most people purchase today at their local grocery store.

However, some animal parts were too tough to chew. Discovering rather quickly that heat would break down the bones and draw out the precious nutrients, our ancestors likely started dropping hot rocks into the carcasses of the animal to heat up the bones and break them down.

The invention of the pot changed things forever. Once people could hang a pot above a fire, they could throw bones into the pot and let it brew for hours. Later, vegetables, tubers, herbs, and spices were added to create a complete meal. The word "bru" is the Germanic root of bone broth and means to "prepare for boiling."

Used as a natural healer for millennia, just about every culture throughout history has used a form of bone broth to improve health. Traditional Chinese meals use a light soup made from bones and vegetables. A Korean dish, seolleongtang, uses ox bones and brisket. The Japanese eat a noodle soup (tonkotsu) made with pork bones. In Greece, Hippocrates recommended it to people with digestive issues. Maimonides, a Medieval philosopher of Judaism, recommended chicken bone broth as an excellent food and medication. This may explain why chicken soup is sometimes called "Jewish penicillin." Caribbean people know it as "cow foot soup" and eat it as a healthy breakfast. South Americans claim that "good bone broth can resurrect the dead."

Rich in minerals, amino acids, protein, collagen, and gelatin, this amazing superfood has immense benefits:

- **Promotes weight loss** - good source of L-glutamine (gut health)
- **Restores exercise capacity** - rehydrates with quality electrolytes
- **Look younger** - rich in collagen for hair, skin, and nails
- **Reduces inflammation** - contains glucosamine and chondroitin sulfate
- **Sleep better** - high in glycine for improved sleep
- **Improves digestion** - helps with the growth of probiotics
- **Stronger bones and teeth** - rich in phosphorus, magnesium, and calcium
- **Protects joints** - high in glucosamine and chondroitin
- **Boosts immunity** - rich in amino acids (arginine, glutamine, and cysteine)

- **Heal and seal gut** - contains gelatin that helps seal holes in the intestines
- **Economical** - bones, veggies, and herbs don't break the bank

For the healthiest and easiest bone broth, use only organic bones: knuckles, necks, oxtails, and soup bones. Grandma's chicken soup really was a healer after all!

"The doctor of the future will no longer
treat the human frame with drugs,
but will cure and prevent disease with nutrition."
~ Thomas Edison, American inventor and businessman

Drinking red wine daily can help you live longer and lose weight.

Fact.

Drinking a glass of red wine a day may be the single most important thing you can do from an anti-aging point of view, other than not smoking.

With only 20-calories per ounce, it delivers numerous antioxidants, decreasing the risks of heart disease and increasing HDL levels. According to David Sinclair, a professor of genetics at Harvard Medical School, "In the history of pharmaceuticals, there has never been a drug that binds to a protein to make it run faster in the way that resveratrol activates SIRT1."

SIRT1 is a serum that prevents diseases and slows aging by boosting the energy production in our cells. Resveratrol, a phytoalexin (natural antibiotic) found in grapes, blueberries, and raspberries is responsible for most of the health benefits associated with this ancient drink. Red wine contains a whopping 13:1 ratio of resveratrol over white wine. Malbecs and Pinot Noirs (wine grapes grown in cooler climates) have the highest concentration of resveratrol.

Dating back some 5,400 years, red wine has been a drink of choice for numerous reasons: social, emotional, religious, pleasure, taste, and because it is therapeutic.

Would you believe that drinking red wine can help you lose weight? Surprisingly, two studies by Washington State University and Harvard University show this statement to be true. Scientists have found that resveratrol restricts the conversion of fat cells. Two glasses a day can reduce obesity by up to 70%! A study by the University of Ulm in Germany also shows that resveratrol inhibits preadipocytes (the precursors to fat cells) from increasing in size and changing to mature adipocytes. Resveratrol also minimizes fat storage. Maybe this is one reason the French are so lean?

According to University of Rochester Medical Center neuroscientist Dr. Maiken Nedergaard, "Low doses of alcohol are potentially beneficial to the brain, namely it improves the brain's ability to remove waste." Another Harvard study in 2012 found drinking red wine later in the day can help reduce your hunger in the evening.

The many benefits of red wine include:

- Boosts heart health
- Improves cholesterol
- Helps manage diabetes
- Fights free radical damage
- Fights obesity and weight gain
- May help prevent certain cancers
- May help prevent Alzheimer's disease

Experts recommend no more than 6-ounces of red wine per day for women and 12-ounces per day for men. My wife and I enjoy 1-2 glasses (Malbec or Pinot Noir) most evenings with some dark chocolate. I prefer one glass when I get home from work and another with dinner.

"I cook with wine. Sometimes I even add it to the food."
~ W.C. Fields, the late American comedian and actor

Stay away from beer unless you want a beer belly.

Myth.

"In general, alcohol intake is associated with bigger waists, because when you drink alcohol, the liver burns alcohol instead of fat," says Michael Jensen, MD, an endocrine expert and obesity researcher with the Mayo Clinic in Rochester, Minnesota. Alcohol calories are easy to overdo, whether from beer, wine, or liquor. A typical beer has 150-calories. Having a few beers in one sitting can increase caloric intake quickly.

Beer can increase your appetite, so the foods that are washed down with beer add even more calories. Typically, these foods are empty calories from unhealthy foods, like pizza, French fries, or chicken wings. All this equals a rounder mid-section.

Our fat storage is determined by our sex, age, and hormones. Girls and boys start out with similar fat storage patterns, but that changes with puberty. Women have more subcutaneous (under the skin) fat than men, deposited in the thighs, butt, and arms, as well as the belly. Men have less subcutaneous fat, typically stored in their bellies.

The all too popular beer belly is more common in older folks. As you get older, you often become less active, your caloric needs go down, and fat is stored more easily. With hormone levels dropping as they age, women and men are more likely to store fat around the midsection.

Belly fat is linked to many health problems, including high blood pressure, diabetes, and cardiovascular disease. The fat that you carry around the abdominal cavity is much more dangerous than that found on your butt, thighs, and hips.

"When waist circumference exceeds 35-inches for women and 40-inches for men, it is associated with an increased risk of heart disease, metabolic syndrome, and overall mortality," Jensen says. He cautions that these numbers are simply guidelines, and recommends keeping your waist size well below these numbers.

With an explosion of small breweries across the U.S, we now have over 3,000 microbreweries in America.

Microbrews have several advantages over the big breweries:

- Since they are made in smaller batches with better ingredients they have a better flavor from the quality of the hops to the fresh berries in some.
- Why drink an industrial light beer if it tastes like crap?
- Being more satisfying, you drink less. This equals less alcohol, carbs and calories.
- They often go hand in hand with great food.
- You're supporting small businesses.
- Healthier for the gut since they contain microbes.

Contrary to popular belief, stouts can have the lowest calories, lowest alcohol content, and can be the lightest in body. Many people believe dark beers are heavy, rich, and full of calories. This is not always the case. The color of the beer is directly related to its malt content. Don't fear the dark!

If you have not tried local craft beers, I highly recommend them. Try a flight (numerous small glasses, each with a different style of beer) with a friend or by yourself to see what you like. There is an endless array of flavors.

Drink local. Eat local. Drink and eat responsibly!

"The University of Nebraska says that elderly people that drink beer or wine at least four times a week have the highest bone density. They need it - they're the ones falling down the most."
~ Jay Leno, American comedian, actor, writer, and television host

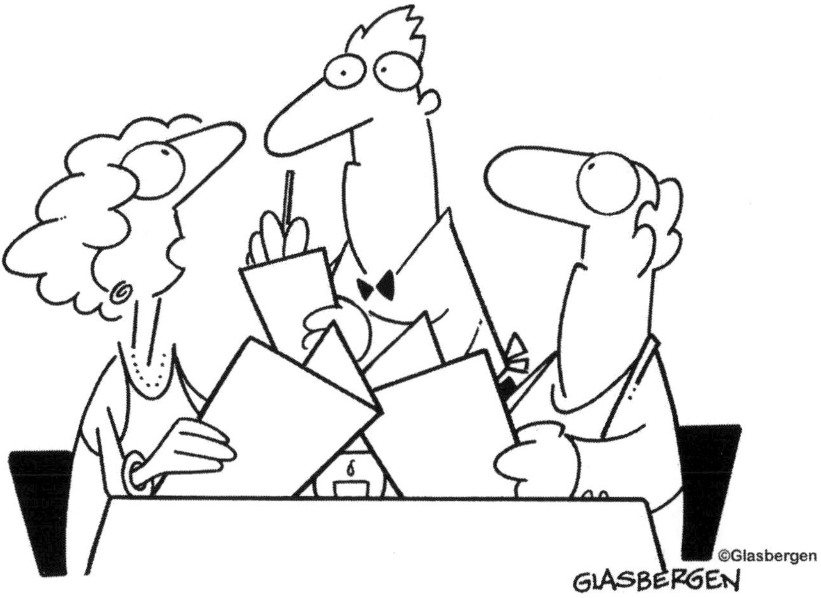

"I would like prime rib with asparagus. My husband would like a bottle of beer, a bag of potato chips and a television."

Intermittent fasting is a fad and has no proven benefits.

Myth.

Eating too much food can be just as bad for the brain as it is for the body.

According to Mark Mattson, Professor of Neuroscience at the Johns Hopkins School of Medicine and Chief of the Laboratory of Neurosciences at the National Institute of Aging, intermittent fasting may help the brain fight off neurodegenerative diseases like Parkinson's Disease and Alzheimer's Disease, while improving mood and memory. Intermittent fasting is the cycle between periods of eating and fasting. Typically done for 16-24 hours, one-to-three days a week.

Mattson's research has spanned decades on caloric intake and brain function. Intermittent fasting can help improve neural connections in the hippocampus and protect neurons against the accumulation of amyloid plaques, a protein found in people with Alzheimer's Disease.

"Fasting is a challenge to the brain, and we think that your brain reacts by activating adaptive stress responses that help it cope with disease," says Mattson. "From an evolutionary perspective, it makes sense your brain should be functioning well when you haven't been able to obtain food for a while."

But what if you just don't eat as much? It's not that simple. Every time you eat, glucose is stored in your liver (becoming glycogen), which takes 10-12 hours to be depleted. After glycogen, fat is burned and converted into ketone bodies, which are acidic chemicals used by neurons for energy. These ketones promote positive changes in synapses that are responsible for memory, learning, and brain health.

Mattson suggests starting off with one-day per-week of moderate fasting and then progressing to two or three. Try to fast for 16-24 hours from your last meal (i.e.: dinner at 7:00 pm on Saturday and fast until 1:00 pm on Sunday). You may experience headaches, lightheadedness, and grogginess for the first week or two.

According to another expert, Dr. Jason Fung, a Canadian nephrologist, intermittent fasting may actually reverse aging by getting the junk (old cellular matter) out and replacing it with new cells. All the junk is responsible for the aging process. We must get rid of the old before putting in the new. It's like rebuilding a car: the old parts need to be scrapped before putting in the new ones. The destruction is just as important as the creation.

Benefits from intermittent fasting:

- **Changes the functions of hormones**. Insulin levels drop and fat burning starts. An increase of HGH (by as much as 5 fold) burns fat and builds muscle.
- **Changes the functions of cells and genes**. Cell repair helps remove waste material. Change in genes help with longevity and disease prevention.
- **Increases in metabolism** by 3-14%, helping to burn fat.

- **Reduces insulin resistance** lowering type 2 diabetes. A 20-31% decrease in fasting insulin has been documented.
- **Reduces oxidative stress and inflammation**
- **Helps cellular repair** by removing metabolized and dysfunctional proteins (autophagy).
- **May decrease heart disease** by decreasing triglycerides in the blood stream.
- **May extend lifespan** with all the known benefits for mental and health markers.
- **May help control hunger** by controlling ghrelin (a hunger hormone).

"Fasting is the single greatest natural healing therapy.
It is nature's ancient, universal 'remedy' for many problems.
Animals instinctively fast when ill."

~ Dr. Elson Haas, M.D., Integrative medicine pioneer and author

Don's Pantry, Fridge and Freezer

Chances are that a significant portion of the food you have in and around your kitchen is compromising your health. It's high time to eliminate these inferior provisions and replace them with nourishing edibles instead. The following items should be the mainstay of the choices found in your cupboards as well as that big cold box in your kitchen:

Pantry items:

- Almond extract
- Almond flour
- Apple cider vinegar
- Avocado oil
- Avocados
- Baking powder
- Baking soda
- Beans
- Beef liver capsules
- Blackstrap molasses
- Braggs liquid amino acids
- Cacao powder
- Canned green beans
- Canned green chili
- Canned herring fillets (Kipper Snacks)
- Canned oysters
- Canned sardines
- Canned tuna
- Cinnamon
- Coconut flour

- Coconut oil
- Coconut sugar
- Coffee
- Curry
- Dark chocolate
- Dulce
- Flax oil
- Garlic
- Ginger
- Italian seasoning
- Kelp powder
- MCT oil
- Meat sticks
- Millet
- Monk fruit (liquid or powder)
- Multivitamin (food grade)
- Nutmeg
- Nutritional yeast
- Nut butters
- Oats
- Olive oil
- Onions
- Potatoes
- Protein bars (low sugar varieties)
- Quinoa
- Raw honey
- Red wine
- Rice
- Rice pasta
- Roasted seaweed
- Sea salt
- Seed butters
- Stevia

- Teas
- Teff
- Vanilla extract
- Whey protein powder (hormone-free; organic when possible)
- Yams

Fridge/freezer items:

Vegetables: (organic, local, and fresh when possible; frozen, if necessary)

- Artichokes
- Arugula
- Asparagus
- Beans
- Beets
- Broccoli
- Brussel sprouts
- Cabbage
- Carrots
- Cauliflower
- Celery
- Chard
- Collard greens
- Eggplant
- Fennel
- Kale
- Mushrooms (technically a fungus)
- Peas
- Radishes
- Spinach
- Zucchini

Meats and Eggs: (hormone-free, nitrate-free, grass-fed choices when possible)

- Bacon
- Beef
- Chicken
- Deli meat
- Eggs
- Fish
- Hot dogs
- Lamb
- Pork
- Sausage
- Turkey

Nuts/Seeds:

- Almonds
- Brazil nuts
- Cashews
- Flax seeds
- Hazelnuts
- Hemp seeds
- Macadamia nuts
- Pecans
- Pumpkin seeds
- Sunflower seeds
- Walnuts

Dairy: (hormone-free, grass-fed, full-fat choices when possible)

- Butter
- Cheese (cow, goat)
- Cottage cheese

- Ghee
- Greek yogurt (plain)
- Heavy whipping cream (for coffee & desserts)
- Ricotta cheese

Fruits: (low-moderate glycemic)

- Apples
- Bell peppers (technically a fruit)
- Berries
- Cherries
- Cucumbers (technically a fruit)
- Grapes
- Prunes
- Tomatoes (technically a fruit)

Condiments: (low-to-no sugar varieties)

- Earth Balance (vegetarian spread)
- Horseradish (raw)
- Ketchup
- Lemon juice
- Lime juice
- Mayonnaise
- Mustard
- Salsa
- Sauerkraut
- Sriracha

Grains:

- Bread (gluten-free, sourdough or sprouted is best)
- Tortillas (same)

Drinks:

- Almond milk (unsweetened)
- Coconut milk (unsweetened)
- Cow's milk (whole; hormone-free)
- Craft beer
- Dry hard cider (has very little sugar)
- Tea (unsweetened)
- Stevia sweetened soda

Other:

- Almond cheese (high protein, vegan)
- Tempeh (high protein, fermented soy)

Use the choices above as a grocery shopping list.

"If all else fails, pillage the fridge."
~ Rene Gutteridge, award-winning and best-selling author

A Don Story: Grand Canyon Cuisine

It was Spring Break 2016, and we were heading to the Grand Canyon, a chasm so vast, it may best be appreciated by hiking. My family of four, along with our friend's family of four, would be spending several days at the bottom of the canyon. Having hiked down the Bright Angel Trail (the flat, wide, and popular one that the majority of tourists use) in 1985 as a senior in high school, I knew a little about the magnitude of such a feat. This trip, however, would be very different from thirty-plus years ago.

First and foremost, we would be on a rugged, narrow, and remote trail that makes the Bright Angel Trail seem like a walk in the park. In addition, we would be carrying large backpacks, which weren't part of my high school endeavor. We only did a day hike with water and snacks back then.

Doing a mock setup with our camping gear at our home the night before, we felt confident in the necessities that we'd be carrying. Tents, sleeping bags, air mattresses, clothes, a mini-stove, water bottles, and a water filter were fitting nicely with plenty of room for grub.

Having much more experience in hiking than we did, our friends offered to do all of the food prep for the journey. We were pleased they had offered, since we weren't privy to appropriate hiking food for eight people. The copious rations would be divvied-up once we began our descent.

Arriving at the canyon the evening before the big day, we camped on the rim to minimize driving time to the trailhead, which was only a few miles away.

Waking with great anticipation, we gathered for coffee and breakfast while discussing food distribution. With eight moderate-to-large sized backpacks placed in a large circle, the items were handed off fairly quickly.

With our backpacks stuffed and our adrenaline running high, we loaded our two vehicles and made the short drive to the trailhead. It was a perfect day for hiking, with the temperatures in the 60's and clouds overhead.

Doing a quick checklist and saying a prayer, we loaded the packs onto our backs and began the eight-mile four-thousand-foot descent. Even though my pack felt unusually heavy, I assumed it was normal since I hadn't had a big pack on in roughly twenty years. Fortunately, we stopped every hour or so to take a break and grab a snack. It felt like I had been carrying my oldest son piggyback! He weighed 90-pounds at the time. I estimated the fathers were each carrying roughly 80-pounds, the mothers 60-pounds, and the kids 40-pounds.

About four hours into the hike we were only halfway (four miles and two thousand feet) to our destination. Removing our packs, we took a long (30-minute) break and had a huge snack and water. Cheese, nuts, and chocolate were the chosen provisions. These certainly weren't the lightest edibles to bring, but they were definitely calorie dense. As we finished our much needed break, I glanced at some of the other items in our packs. Two large cans of spaghetti sauce were showing their labels. Holy crap! At 32-ounces a piece, these weighed 8 pounds. How did I miss these when packing? What else are we carrying in these packs? I scratched my head in wonder, loaded my pack and we pushed on.

With my shoulders and right knee feeling pretty uncomfortable, it was as though we had been walking for twice as long as we actually had. Built in 1911, this rocky, steep, and strenuous route was the most extreme I had encountered in my lifetime. Little did I know, the most difficult part, the infamous Cathedral Stairs were still hours ahead.

I suddenly remembered it was Easter weekend. I thought about the insurmountable pain and suffering that Christ had sustained. If he could endure the torture of being flogged while carrying an enormous cross, then we could certainly overcome this.

Having my two boys in view ahead, my wife struggling far behind, and being afraid of heights, this only added to my anxiety that had built for hours. "What the hell are we doing on such an extreme trail?"

Hours later, as we approached the top of the Cathedral Staircase, we took another long break and indulged in more snacks. This time the choice was energy squares - full of peanut butter, honey, and other high calorie ingredients. Fatigued and thirsty, we savored every morsel of food and drop of water. Even though we were eating some of the heavy food items from the packs and drinking a few quarts of water, it didn't seem to lighten the load, as we were on the brink of exhaustion.

I felt like a 260-pound, biped pack mule (weighing 180 pounds plus 80 pounds on my back) as I carefully chose each step down the brutally tough descent of the staircase. With gravel, small boulders, and a narrow valley, navigating through the tight switchbacks was the toughest part of the seven hours we had been hiking. I thought of Christ again and how brutally he was tortured. This was nothing compared to that. We'll get through this, I kept affirming to myself.

On the verge of collapsing, we pushed on. At one point, my wife stated that it was tougher than bearing children, which she had endured for more than 12 hours with each of our boys!

Finally, around another bend, we could see our campsite below. Judging by the distance, it appeared to only be 20-30 minutes away. I was way off, as it took another hour to reach. The immensity of the canyon can fool the eye.

With the sun starting to set and unable to take another step, we pitched camp.

Blistered feet, sore backs, aching muscles, a sprained ankle, and a bum knee made the list for injuries. Most of us were on the verge of passing out, but we had made it to the bottom of what must be one of the most difficult trails on the planet. We had conquered the dragon!

For the next three days, we ate like royalty. Hauling a few dozen scrambled eggs in Nalgene bottles, we made omelets for most breakfasts. For snacks, we devoured pounds of nuts, seeds, and nut-butter energy nuggets. Lunches consisted of either ham and cheese or peanut butter and jelly sandwiches. Dinners were either pasta with real spaghetti sauce (remember the two big cans?) or pizzas, made with tortillas and cheese. We certainly had enough food. Hell, we had enough for a dozen people or more. In fact, on the day we departed, we left about twenty pounds of extra rations in a marked spot for other hikers to consume.

Leaving a day early, due to poor weather, I led our group up and out of the Cathedral Staircase and beyond. Hiking uphill was easier on the knees and the rest of the body. Of course, we each had about 20-30 less pounds strapped to our backs.

The upward journey took just as long, about eight hours, but with cooler temperatures than our descent and knowing what lay ahead, we had a little more spring in our step. We also had a meal and margaritas waiting for us at a local Mexican restaurant in the Canyon Village, not to mention a shower and a bed.

The views throughout this wild adventure were simply breathtaking and the solitude was incredibly peaceful. If it hadn't been for the cool temperatures and the sheer beauty, I'm not sure we would have made it.

If you've never experienced the Grand Canyon, I highly recommend it.

However, I have a few critical pieces of advice:

- Wear the best hiking shoes and clothes you can afford.
- Hike only in the spring or fall, as the summer is dangerously hot.
- Pack all of your own gear, including food. Make damn sure that most of that food is dehydrated or at least lightweight.

"Ounces leads to pounds, pounds leads to pain!"
~ U.S. Marine Corps saying

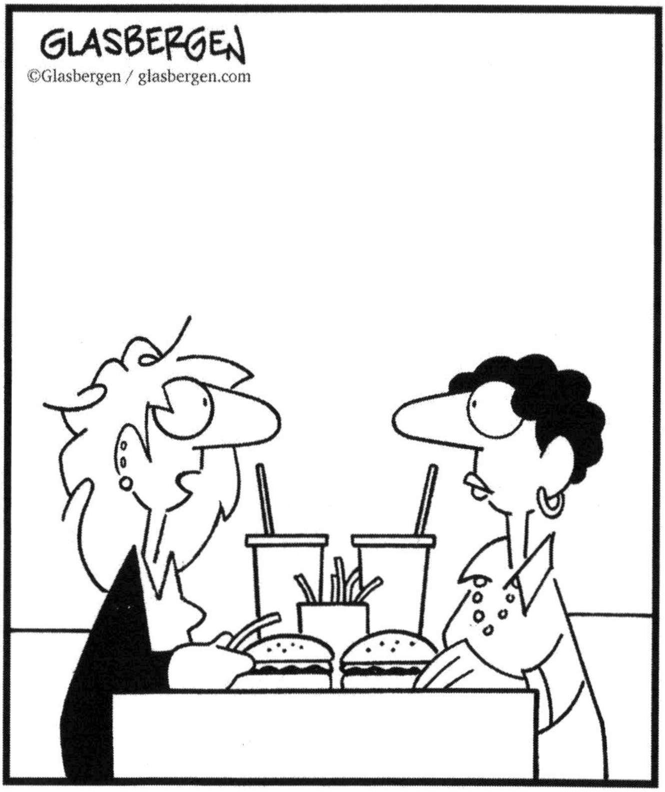

"Unfortunately, I have one pair of running shoes and sixteen pairs of eating shoes!"

Don's Tips for Controlling Food Consumption

- Eat slowly
- Eat mindfully
- Chew thoroughly
- Spice up your meals
- Eat more fiber and fat
- Drink out of a tall glass
- Eat outdoors if possible
- Eat away from your desk
- Start with a salad or soup
- Place fruit on the counter
- Drink water between meals
- Make half your plate veggies
- Use your non-dominant hand
- Eat protein at every meal/snack
- Use small plates, forks, and spoons
- Choose soft light/slow music while eating
- Keep junk food out of sight and out of your house
- Eat whole foods and avoid food from a box or bag

"Appetite has really become an artificial and abnormal thing, having taken the place of true hunger, which alone is natural. The one is a sign of bondage, but the other, of freedom."
~ Paul Brunton, British theosophist and spiritualist

Don's Food Pyramid (Non-traditional)

Sugar
Juice, Soda
Refined Grains
Bread, Cereal, Pasta
Alcoholic Beverages
Beer, Red Wine, Vodka
High-Glycemic Fruits
Bananas, Melons, Pineapple
Whole Grains
Buckwheat, Millet, Oats, Quinoa, Rice
Low-Glycemic Fruits
Apples, Berries, Cherries, Grapefruit, Peaches
Starchy Vegetables
Beets, Beans, Legumes, Peas, Pumpkin, Squash, Yams
Fruit and Vegetable Fats
Avocado, Avocado Oil, Coconut, Coconut Oil, Olives, Olive Oil
Nuts, Nut Butters, Seeds, Seed Butters
Almonds, Almond Butter, Flax Seeds, Pumpkin Seeds, Tahini, Walnuts
Animal Proteins and Fats
Beef, Chicken, Cow/Goat Cheeses, Eggs, Fish, Lamb, Turkey, Wild Game
Fibrous Vegetables
Asparagus, Broccoli, Cabbage, Cauliflower, Celery, Kale, Onions, Spinach

"Traditional food pyramids show how food and agriculture institutions can exert lobbying and political power on the USDA to feature and prioritize the subsidizing of industries like corn, dairy and wheat."

~ **Marion Nestle, professor of nutrition at New York University, author of *Food Politics***

Don's Nutrition Tips and Reminders

- Mainly eat protein, fat, and fiber since they curb the appetite. Quick absorbing carbs (juice, cereal, bread, crackers, etc.) make you fat, tired and hungry.
- Minimize or eliminate sugar and flour. They both suppress the immune system, making us more vulnerable to disease.
- Combine fibrous vegetables with fats and proteins as much as possible. Starches (like quick absorbing carbs) combined with protein can make digestion more difficult.
- "Low-fat" foods are absorbed too fast and they minimize absorption of vitamins A, E, D, and K. Eat whole-fat foods.
- We are designed to eat vegetables, nuts, seeds, fish, meat, fruit, some dairy, and minimal grains/flour.
- Shop mainly the "perimeter" of the grocery store. Center isles contain more refined foods.
- Eat one to two "treat meals" (anything) weekly, this will keep you from binging.
- Rotate your foods to help prevent food allergies, to help maximize nutrient absorption, and so you don't get tired of them.
- Weigh yourself once a week (at most), upon waking. Your health, strength, and how you feel and look are most important.

- Use stevia, monk fruit, coconut sugar, or a little raw honey instead of artificial sweeteners. Avoid Sucralose, Aspartame, Splenda, etc.
- Drink yerba mate and/or green tea on a regular basis. Both are super healthy.
- Drink organic coffee (black or with real cream) and/or MCT oil.
- Coconut milk ice cream is a tasty, non-dairy option, but it still has a fair amount of sugar.
- *Amy's* Rice Crust pizza, *Against the Grain* GF pizza, or *Udi's* GF crust with added meat and/or veggies are all gluten-free options, but generally avoid eating food that comes in a box!
- "A calorie is a calorie." Not so! A pancake and an egg have the same calories: the pancake triggers different hormones than the egg and will make you feel hungry, tired, and store fat.
- Use these health-promoting herbs regularly: curry, ginger, cinnamon, cayenne, turmeric, garlic, oregano, rosemary, and thyme.
- The "best of the worst" fast foods: Wendy's Chili; Subway salad
- Dark chocolate (70-90%) is a nice treat (low sugar) and contains healthy antioxidants.
- Salsa, horseradish, hummus, and mustard are great for flavor and have little to no carbs or sugar (but read the label).
- It takes 3-4 weeks to develop a new habit. Make it a mission to eat a nutritious diet and exercise regularly.
- Beware of the three "white devils": white sugar, white flour, and iodized salt. Use these healthy alternatives instead: stevia, monk fruit, or RAW

honey (small amount), almond or coconut (gluten-free) flour, and sea salt.

- Fermented foods, like sauerkraut, kimchi, and kombucha (low sugar variety) are wonderful for your gut flora. Eat them regularly.
- Unless you are eating lots of fermented veggies, take a probiotic daily.
- Take a quality multi-vitamin daily (preferably food-based).
- Eating smaller amounts (2-3 meals, plus 2-3 snacks) roughly every 3-4 hours is like putting kindling on a fire (food will digest easier and your metabolism will boost). For most people this will also minimize or eliminate over-eating.
- Garlic, oregano oil, and olive leaf extract are all natural antibiotics to fight-off the most stubborn of bacteria and viruses.
- Celtic sea salt contains most of the minerals we need in perfect balance. Eat it daily.
- Pay now (money) or pay later (health): Choose organic, hormone-free, local, whole foods when possible.
- Fast 1-2 days per-week to increase human growth hormone and regenerate cell growth. Fasting 16-24 hours works well.
- Use a nutrition journal to keep track of your progress and record your emotions.
- Don't beat yourself up if you have a bad day of eating poorly. Get back on track the next day and do your best. You control your own destiny.

"Trust the process: Eat clean. Be patient. Work hard."

~ Unknown

Section Four

Other Health Myths and Facts

Sleep is more important than exercise and nutrition.

Fact.

Shocking evidence from the *Annals of Internal Medicine* shows that the lack of sleep is absolutely killing people's metabolism.

Side effects of inadequate sleep are:

- **You look and feel older.** Sleep deprivation restricts the production of growth hormones, which are the primary "youth" hormones that work their magic when you sleep. Have you ever noticed how much older people look when they are sleep deprived?
- **You feel super hungry with increased cravings for junk food**. The *Public Library of Science* shows that leptin (feel full) hormone decreases by up to 15.5% when you get inadequate sleep. Ghrelin (hunger) hormone increases by up to 14.9% when sleep is impaired. You wake up starving and feeling useless, until you binge on poor foods. Lack of sleep gets you addicted to the worst

foods, increases cravings for sugar, sweets, breads, pastas, etc.

- **Your cognitive abilities and mood are impaired**. Sleep allows your brain to flush out potent neurotoxins. Brain fog, impaired memory, mood swings, and trouble focusing are all signs of inadequate sleep.
- **Your sensitivity to insulin is increased**. We must increase sleep to clear the blood sugar from the bloodstream. Lack of sleep increases insulin, doubling the fat that your body is producing; lack of sleep tells the liver to turn the food you eat into fat and to lock fat in your fat cells. The body perceives lack of sleep to be a threat, so it increases cortisol (stress hormones), which is directly linked to belly fat.

In addition, lack of sleep can play a vital role in car accidents. In 2009, the National Highway Traffic Safety Administration reported that being tired accounted for the highest number of fatal, single-car, run-off-the-road crashes.

Fifty-to-seventy million Americans have sleep disorders. *Forbes Magazine* states that 60-million Americans filled prescriptions for sleeping pills in 2012; up from 46 million in 2006.

According to Matt Walker, a professor of neuroscience and psychology at the University of California, Berkeley, sleep medications don't deliver the same restorative benefits as natural sleep. In fact, the research shows that drugs don't increase sleep quality any better than placebos. Psychological methods are superior to pharmacological ones.

Tips for falling asleep include:

- **Eliminating devices.** Turn off your smart phones, computers, TVs, etc., within 3-hours of bedtime. These devices overstimulate the mind, making it much harder to fall asleep. Try reading a book. The more boring, the better.
- **Drink no caffeine after midday**. It takes roughly 6-hours to process and eliminate caffeine. If you have adrenal fatigue, consider eliminating caffeine all together.
- **Eat cherries or drink tart cherry juice at bedtime**. Cherries contain melatonin. You can also add cherry juice or cherry juice concentrate to herbal tea at night.
- **Don't overdose on melatonin supplements**. Most supplements are 3-5 milligrams, which is too much. Overdosing on melatonin makes it hard to wake up and disrupts the sleep pattern for the next night. One milligram or less is best.
- **Drink night-time teas.** Chamomile, mint, lemongrass (or all mixed) are excellent choices. The side benefit of chamomile is that it has unique phytonutrients that fight estrogenic overload from chemicals and pesticides, which we are all exposed to in various ways and amounts.
- **Take magnesium.** Magnesium is known to calm the nervous system and help with insomnia and anxiety. Taken 30-minutes before bed can be very beneficial. A powdered form called, "Calm," is what my wife and I use.

Several studies confirm that houseplants can also help with insomnia, allergies, stress; they also remove toxins, and promote drowsiness. Sleep better with these plants in the bedroom:

- **Jasmine** - Similar to barbiturates, eases anxiety and encourages sleep
- **Lavender** - Bouquets and essential oils are sleep inducers
- **Aloe Vera** – Vacuums up unhealthy indoor chemicals
- **English Ivy** - Helps clear the air of mold spores, keeping the air clean
- **Boston Fern** - Removes formaldehyde from the air
- **Snake Plant** - An air cleaner that is simple to care for

If you need an alarm clock to wake-up, you're not getting enough sleep! A national panel of sleep experts recommends the following amounts of sleep:

- Older Adults (65+ years) 7-8 hours
- Adults (18 - 64) 7-9 hours
- Teenagers (14 - 18) 8-10 hours
- School Age Children (6-13 years) 9-11 hours
- Preschoolers (3-5 years) 10-13 hours
- Toddlers (1-2 years) 11-14 hours
- Infants (4-11 months) 12-15 hours
- Newborns (0-3 months) 14-17 hours

"Muscles are torn in the gym, fed in the kitchen, and built in the bed." ~ **Unknown**

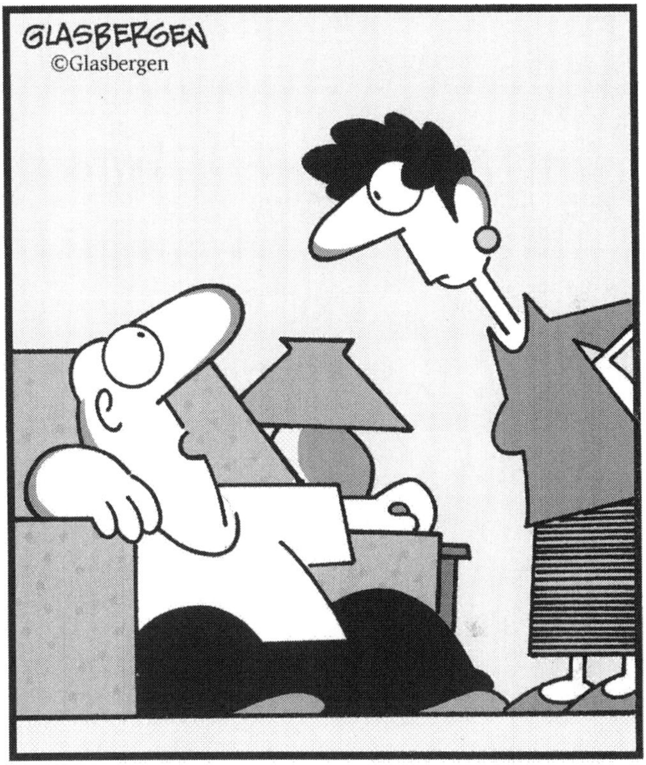

"Napping is the best activity for weight loss. I can't eat anything when I'm asleep!"

Our gut-brain connection is closely linked.

Fact.

What's going on in your gut could be affecting your brain, and vice versa. If you've ever felt "butterflies in your stomach" when nervous or "gone with your gut" to make a decision, you are probably getting signals from your *second* brain. Lying in the walls of your digestive system, this "brain in your gut" is transforming medicine's understanding of the connection between mood, digestion, health, and even the way you think. Anxiety, anger, sadness, elation - all of these feelings (and more) can generate symptoms in the gut.

Just thinking about eating releases digestive juices before food gets there and a troubled intestine can send signals to the brain. It is difficult to heal a distressed gut without considering stress and other emotions.

Called the enteric nervous system (ENS), this second brain comprises more than 100 million nerve cells lining your gastrointestinal tract from esophagus to rectum. Incapable of making decisions like our big brain, the main role of the ENS is controlling digestion. "The enteric nervous system doesn't seem capable of thought as we know it, but it communicates back and forth with our big brain-with profound results," says Jay Pasricha, M.D., director of the Johns Hopkins Center for Neurogastroenterology, whose research has gathered international attention.

A new scientific study from the University of Cambridge reveals that changes in the microbiome (gut bacteria) may control many aspects of human health. Our gut bacteria actually outnumbers our cells by a staggering factor of 10 to one. With 40 trillion bacteria in the body, most are in the intestines. Unfortunately, things like antibiotics and chlorinated water, deplete our microbiome. The foods you eat greatly affect the health of your gut and subsequently your brain.

Science-based ways to improve your gut bacteria:

- **Eat a variety of foods**. There are hundreds of different species of bacteria in your gut, with each requiring different nutrients. The more species of bacteria you have, the greater the health benefits. A diet rich in whole foods establishes better gut health.
- **Eat lots of vegetables, beans, legumes, and fruit**. High in fiber, these foods stimulate gut bacteria growth.
- **Eat fermented foods**. Fermenting typically involves yeasts or bacteria converting the sugars in food to organic acids or alcohol. Sauerkraut, kimchi, tempeh, kombucha, yogurt, and kefir are all examples. Choose low sugar varieties.
- **Don't eat artificial sweeteners**. Some studies have shown they negatively affect gut health.
- **Eat whole grains**. Foods like quinoa, oats, millet, barley, spelt, brown rice, teff, rye, and others promote healthy intestinal bacteria.
- **Eat foods rich in polyphenols**. These are plant compounds with many health benefits, including reductions in cholesterol, inflammation, blood pressure, and oxidative stress. Almonds, blueberries, broccoli, dark chocolate, grapes, green tea, and red wine are all good sources.

- **Take a probiotic supplement when ill**. These live microorganisms temporarily help to colonize our gut with bacteria. In sick people, this can be beneficial. However, a review of seven studies found that probiotic supplements have little effect on the guts of healthy individuals.

"Every day we live and every meal we eat,
we influence the great microbial organ inside us -
for better or for worse."
~ **Giulia Enders, German scientist and author, *Gut, 2014***

Food cravings are mostly due to our emotional state.

Fact.

Research shows that people having trouble identifying emotions are more prone to overeat. We are temporarily fulfilled and comforted by the foods that we eat. Sweet, salty, spicy, and sour food cravings all play an interesting role in our emotions. Understanding these cravings may shed some light on those emotions. For thousands of years, Chinese medicine has correlated food, mood, and organ systems together.

Why we crave these foods:

- **Sweet** - is our first taste from breastfeeding our mother's milk. It is the most frequent craving that people admit to and includes all carbohydrates. Craving sweets can be a sign of low energy; eating them gives a quick high and then a big low, causing us to crave more sugar. Sweetness relates to an emotion of disconnection and/or abandonment; people who crave sweets may be lacking joy in their life. If this is the case, it is important to get your blood sugar into balance.
- **Salty -** involves the kidneys, adrenal glands, and water balance. Our kidneys are our water filter. The emotions of fear and anxiety deplete our kidneys both energetically and physiologically, causing stress and tightness, which may lead to low back pain, anxiety, intense thirst and

hypertension, coldness, poor memory, impotence, premature graying, and frequent urination. Consuming excess salt (especially the regular iodized variety) leads to rigidity of the mind and body. The brands Celtic, Himalayan, and Real Salt are all great choices and are far superior to the bleached, iodized type. Be sure to stay hydrated by drinking roughly half your bodyweight in ounces of water daily.

- **Spicy** - is considered lung energy. Feelings of grief or loss can be associated with spicy food cravings. A lung problem may show up as a cough, body aches, excess sweating, allergy symptoms or difficulty breathing. Chinese medicine associates foods like garlic, ginger, onions, and pepper with the lungs. Wanting spicy food may be a craving for more intensity and action in one's life. Spicy foods tend to rev the imagination and our ability to be intuitive.
- **Sour -** calms the mind and body and is considered liver (our giant filter) energy. Emotions of depression and anger can be associated with sour foods. Tart foods like pickles, lemons, and apple cider vinegar are all good choices when you crave something sour.

"You can't fight cravings simply with a strong will because it will keep you stuck in a never-ending battle with yourself. It's too draining. Over time your will fades and you lose."
~ Laura Hussein, American actor

Fluoride is safe for drinking water.

Myth.

The addition of fluoride to public drinking water supplies is a controversial health topic to say the least; the benefits and harms of which have been debated since its introduction in the U.S.

In 1945, Grand Rapids, Michigan became the first community in the world to add fluoride to tap water. Initial studies showed much lower rates of cavities in school children, and so water fluoridation spread across the country.

The U.S. Centers for Disease Control named fluoridation one of the 10 great public health achievements of the 20th century. Now many experts question the scientific basis for the intervention.

In 2015, the Cochrane Collaboration, a global independent network of healthcare professionals and researchers, known for meticulous scientific reviews of public health policies, published an analysis of 20 crucial studies on water fluoridation. They concluded that early scientific studies on fluoridation (most were conducted before 1975) were deeply flawed. Countries that do not fluoridate their water have also seen drops in the cavity rates.

While 70% of the U.S. fluoridates public drinking supplies, most modernized nations actually ban fluoride from their drinking water. Austria, Belgium, China, Denmark, Finland, Germany, Hungary, Israel, Norway, and the Netherlands all refuse to use it for consumption. The U.S. is one of the only developed countries that fluoridate their citizens' drinking water.

Sodium fluoride, used in most municipal water, is a waste product of the phosphate fertilizer industry. It is heavily contaminated with toxins and heavy metals (cancerous arsenic, lead, and cadmium), and radioactive materials like radium. These substances accumulate in the human body and are all carcinogens. Sodium fluoride is a byproduct of aluminum, steel, cement, and nuclear weapons. It is used as both a pesticide and herbicide; to refine gasoline; make fluorocarbons and chlorofluorocarbons for air conditioning; and to manufacture computer screens and plastics.

"Residents of cities that fluoridate have double the fluoride in their hip bones vis-a-vis the balance of the population. Worse, we discovered that fluoride is actually altering the basic architecture of human bones," wrote Dr. Hardy Limeback, BS, PhD Biochemistry, DDS, head of Preventative Dentistry at University of Toronto, Canada, President of the Canadian Association for Dental Research. He was once a proponent of fluoridation.

Skeletal fluorosis is a debilitating condition that happens when fluoride accumulates in bones, making them very weak and brittle. In Canada, they are now spending more money treating dental fluorosis than treating cavities.

Toronto, Canada has been fluoridating its drinking water for 50+ years, yet has a higher cavity rate than Vancouver, which does not fluoridate!

Cavity rates are low all across the industrialized world, including Europe, which is 90% fluoride free. The rates are low because of regular dental check-ups, flossing and frequent brushing, and improved standards of living. The World Health Organization's data from 1970-2010 states that in non-fluoridated and fluoridated countries, tooth decay rates of 12-year-olds declined at the same rate.

The intake of fluoride has never been tested for safety on humans! Children and adults who use fluoride toothpastes, mouthwashes, gels, and supplements are far exceeding the recommended intake. The warning on the labels of these items states to, "Call Poison Control if Ingested!" This is mind-blowing, blind-eyed logic for sure.

"If this stuff gets into the air, it's a pollutant; if it gets into a river it's a pollutant; if it gets into a lake, it's a pollutant; if it gets into our drinking water, it's not. That's amazing!" said Dr. William Hirzy, an EPA scientist.

The 60-year history of fluoridation in U.S. cities is an interesting one for sure. Executive action, by local governments, took over and communities had no idea what was happening. After more than half a century of delusion, the CDC, American Dental Association, and Dental Public Health stubbornly and cleverly continue to deceive public opinion in favor of fluoridation.

Reasons to oppose fluoridation of drinking water:

- May lower I.Q.
- Damages bone
- May damage the brain
- May cause bone cancer
- Affects thyroid function
- Dose can't be controlled
- Accumulates in the body
- Not an essential nutrient

- Causes arthritic symptoms
- Numerous scientists oppose
- Benefit is topical not systemic
- May cause reproductive problems
- May cause non-I.Q. neurotoxic effects
- Key health studies have not been done
- May increase hip fractures in the elderly
- No randomized controlled trials for safety
- Children are being overexposed to fluoride
- May increase lead uptake into children's blood
- Other sources of fluoride exist (use toothpaste)
- Proponents use very dubious tactics to promote
- Endorsements do not represent scientific evidence
- Proponents usually refuse to defend in open debate
- Highest doses of fluoride are going to bottle-fed babies
- Tooth decay does not go up when fluoridation is stopped
- Tooth decay is high in low-income communities that have fluoridated for years
- Goes to everyone, regardless of age, health, or vulnerability
- NIH-funded study on tooth decay found no significant benefit
- Dental fluorosis may be an indicator of wider systemic damage
- No health agency monitoring occurs in fluoridated communities
- Studies that launched fluoridation were methodologically flawed

- Only chemical added to water for the purpose of medical treatment

In North America, water fluoridation has come under increased scrutiny. Since 2010, more than 75 U.S. and Canadian communities have voted to end water fluoridation. Fortunately, more and more people are demanding drinking water that does not expose them to this highly toxic industrial waste.

I have a novel idea... stop eating so much FRIGGING SUGAR! This is the very cause of cavities in the first place. Help get rid of fluoridated water in your community.

"Fluoride has been shown to adversely affect the central nervous system, causing behavioral changes, increased hip fractures, and reproductive problems."

~ Natick Report Research Team
research microbiologist, U.S. Army, Dr. B.J. Gallo;
environmental chemist, J. Kupperschmidt;
Apollo Program project scientist, Dr. N.R. Mancuso;
U.S. Army Natick Research Labs, A. Murray;
molecular biologist, Dr. Strauss

Calcium supplements are crucial for the health of your bones.

Myth.

Calcium pills and powders are some of the most overused supplements on the market today. We were becoming a nation of calcium junkies, but the tide is turning.

A 2011 *British Medical Journal* meta-analysis shocked many with the statement: "Risks outweigh benefits for calcium supplements." The study showed that calcium supplements do more harm than good, causing more cardiovascular problems (heart attacks and stroke than the number of bone fractures they prevent). The seven authors of the study expressed: "Even a small increase in incidence of cardiovascular disease could transition into a large burden of disease in the population." They suggest that a reassessment is warranted of the role that calcium supplements play in the prevention and treatment of osteoporosis. The primary treatment for osteoporosis had been high-dosage calcium supplementation! This was a massive admission of failure.

French scientist, Jean Durlach, warned that the 2:1 ratio of calcium to magnesium was a "never to be exceeded" level. Too much calcium along with too little magnesium can cause kidney stones, arthritis, osteoporosis, and calcification of the arteries, leading to cardiovascular disease, stroke, and heart attack.

According to Dr. Robert Thompson and Kathleen Barnes, co-authors of *The Calcium Lie*, published in 2013, most doctors and consumers believe that bones are made of calcium. Even a basic biochemistry textbook will explain the truth: bones are made of at least a dozen minerals, and we need all of them in the proper proportions to have healthy bones and healthy bodies. Thompson and Barnes say that consuming too much calcium through supplements or food sources can cause a multitude of negative health problems: type 2 diabetes, type 2 hypothyroidism, depression, hypertension, pregnancy problems, obesity, and more.

Because of our depleted agricultural soil, most individuals don't get enough magnesium. One hundred years ago we got roughly 500 mg of magnesium per day and now we are fortunate to get 200 mg per day. The calcium to magnesium ratio is now a staggering 10:1. This is a walking time bomb for heart disease, stroke, and bone health.

To balance out your minerals: add a pinch of sea salt to your meals, eat lots of different vegetables, seeds, nuts, and get adequate exercise.

"Milk is for babies..."

~ Arnold Schwarzenegger, Austrian-American actor, producer, businessman, former professional bodybuilder

Nutritional supplements are expensive and not beneficial if you are eating a balanced diet.

Myth.

Our food choices and the quality of food we eat are arguably the most important factors in our nutritional health. However, a sad fact is that the quality of the soil in the United States has been depleted of many crucial minerals through use of pesticides and herbicides, and other mass-production methods. Commercial fruits and vegetables sold today are not as rich in minerals and vitamins as small scale farms or homegrown produce of the past. Even people with a diet rich in whole foods may not be getting the right nutritional balance. But for people eating an imbalanced diet and not getting adequate amounts of sunshine or sleep, food supplements can be especially beneficial.

There are a handful of nutrients that you are probably lacking:

- **Fish oil:** Most experts agree that if you could only take one supplement, this should be the one. Fish oil contains the fatty acids EPA and DHA, which are part of every human cell. Fatty acids allow for better signaling or messaging between cells, allowing for better fat burning instead of relying strictly on carbohydrates. Insulin sensitivity is also improved by fish oil because it has a high thermic effect, allowing the body to burn more calories following digestion. One study found that men who increased their fish oil intake from half a gram to three grams per day for two-weeks, increased their thermic effect by 51%. Fish oil also helps balance the inflammatory effects caused by eating processed foods that use inferior oils from corn, soy, canola, safflower, sunflower, and cottonseed. The average American consumes 15-times more omega-6 oils found in these inferior oils than the omega-3s found in fish and algae. That 15:1 ratio should be closer to 1:1. Consuming omega-6 and omega-3 oils in equal measure means better hormone balance, less stress, improved cognition, and lower risk of degenerative brain diseases like Alzheimer's. My personal favorite is the lemon flavored Norwegian Cod Liver Oil by Carlson which comes in a dark green bottle.

- **Multivitamin/Mineral**: According to a 2002 review by the *Journal of American Medical Association*, "Most people do not consume an optimal amount of vitamins through diet alone." Many factors are at play in the reasons for our nutrient deficiencies: pesticides and herbicides lower nutritional quality; high yield crops deplete the soil of micronutrients; prescription drug use and chronic stress deplete our bodies of micronutrients. Every vitamin and mineral is involved at some level in carbohydrate metabolism and energy production. When selecting a vitamin, pass on cheap, inferior products that are produced using carbonates, oxides, and sulfates. Check your labels for these inferior ingredients. Instead, purchase ones that use arginate, citrate, glycinate, lysinate, orotate, and taurate.

- **Vitamin D:** Extensive research demonstrates that having adequate vitamin D levels is one of the easiest ways to prevent numerous diseases, optimize body composition, promote long term health, and reduce injuries and illnesses. Studies show that more than 100 million Americans are deficient in this vitamin. "50,000-63,000 individuals in the United States and 19,000 in the UK die prematurely from cancer annually due to insufficient vitamin D," states Dr. John Cannell, physician and founder of the Vitamin D Council. A recent study showed that overweight adults who took vitamin D, along with a strength training program, increased their explosive power significantly more than the group that didn't take the supplement. (See more information on vitamin D in the "Sunshine" section.)
- **Magnesium:** Magnesium, an often overlooked mineral that affects some 325 enzyme systems in the body and controls thousands of chemical reactions. Magnesium has a calming effect on the nervous system, making it an ideal sleep aid; relieves muscle aches and spasms; is a natural antidepressant; and a blood sugar and blood pressure stabilizer. Magnesium also helps digestion by relieving constipation; regulates levels of potassium, calcium, and sodium; important for heart health; helps prevent osteoporosis and helps to prevent migraine headaches. The Medical University of South

Carolina found that 68% of U.S. adults consume less than the RDA recommended dose of magnesium and 19% take in less than half. The Linus Pauling Institute supports the latest RDA standards for magnesium intake (400-420 mg/day for men and 310-320 mg/day for women). I prefer a powdered version called "Calm," I like to take it 30-minutes before bedtime mixed with L-Glutamine powder.

- **Probiotics:** Important for digestion and the GI tract; affect the production of neurotransmitters, allowing for better cognition and motivation; support the growth of anti-inflammatory microflora, promoting reductions in body fat. When participants in a Japanese study increased probiotic intake for four-weeks, they decreased belly fat by 8.2 percent. (See more information on probiotics in separate section.)
- **Glutamine:** Found in both animal and plant protein, this essential amino acid is needed for your body in large amounts. Glutamine promotes digestion, brain health, muscle growth, athletic performance; fights cancer and high blood sugar; aids in memory, focus and concentration.; improves gastrointestinal health; helps heal ulcers and leaky gut; cuts sugar and alcohol cravings.

High levels of stress increase the need for the above nutrients. Vitamins, minerals, and antioxidants work synergistically to help prevent toxicity while supplying necessary nourishment. The best way to know if you are lacking a particular micronutrient is to have your blood tested with a functional medical doctor (one who practices holistic medicine). Remember, the recommended daily amount is not necessarily the optimal amount.

"The supplement industry is the biggest threat
to the pharmaceutical industry."
~ Steven Magee, author
Toxic Health

Meditation is an unproven therapy for mental and physical health.

Myth.

Researchers from Johns Hopkins University conducted 47 trials that demonstrated the positive effectiveness of meditation on the body.

Mindful meditation involves sitting comfortably, bringing your mind's attention to the present without drifting into the past or future. Published in *JAMA Internal Medicine*, mindful meditation can help ease psychological conditions such as anxiety, depression, and pain.

"People with anxiety have a problem dealing with distracting thoughts that have too much power," states Dr. Elizabeth Hoge, a psychologist at the Center for Anxiety and Traumatic Stress Disorders at Massachusetts General Hospital, and Associate Professor of Psychology at Harvard Medical School. "They can't distinguish between a problem-solving thought and a nagging worry that has no benefit."

Some people prefer learning mindful meditation techniques and practicing with groups. Others may prefer an app or a guided recording, like "Headspace" or "Everyday Practices for Everyday Problems" by Dr. Ronald Siegel, Assistant Clinical Professor of Psychology at Harvard Medical School (mindfulness-solution.com).

Meditation can improve brain health and aging by altering biochemical pathways in the brain. It is a great low-cost way to use mindfulness to promote health.

People with chronic illnesses can use meditation to decrease stress and increase acceptance of thoughts, feelings, and the health condition they are facing. Meditation decreases stress and illness by providing short-term relief for hypertension. Studies show meditation decreases inflammation at the genomic level - possibly altering the body's hormonal levels over time. More research is needed, however.

Whether a TV, computer, or cell phone, most people start the day looking at a screen. This puts us in a reactive state rather than focusing on internal gratitude.

Cognitive thinking tends to be best in the late morning. Alertness and concentration increases as body temperature rises.

Here are a few things that can help us focus upon waking:

- A short meditation
- Warm shower
- Foam rolling
- Exercise

Small habits like making the bed or balancing your budget can foster a greater sense of well-being. Starting the day with healthy habits like meditation is key for work performance, mood, and interestingly, verbal use, especially in a customer service or sales oriented job.

"The goal of meditation is not to get rid of thoughts or emotions. The goal is to become more aware of your thoughts and emotions and to learn how to move through them without getting stuck."

~ Dr. Philippe R. Goldin, neuroscientist and associate professor at the Betty Irene Moore School of Nursing at University of California, Davis

A Don Story: Meditation Helps in a Crisis

As our home phone rang loudly around 4:00 am, I thought I was dreaming. It was one of the early morning gym members calling from my 24-hour gym in the basement rental space. Feeling sorry that he had disturbed us, he exclaimed that the sprinklers had just come on inside. This was both alarming and confusing, since there were no sprinklers in the gym.

Springing out of bed, my mind raced as fast as my heart beat. What the hell is going on? I grabbed whatever clothes I could find. Fortunately, they didn't belong to my wife. Jumping into my truck and driving far faster than the legal limit, I called the gentlemen back on my cell to assess the situation. However troubling, some of the details started making a little bit of sense.

With little to no traffic on the highway, the usual 20-minute drive took all of 10-minutes as my right foot stayed heavy against the floor. Arriving at the scene, I saw a large fire truck and several firemen in the parking lot of the two-story structure that housed the gym and three other businesses.

A janitor, who was cleaning the natural food store above the gym, had accidentally started a fire in their kitchen. Smoke from the fire activated all the sprinklers in the grocery store. Finding holes in the floor, hundreds of gallons of water had been showering down into the gym, which was below.

Running across the top level parking lot and down the crooked metal outdoor stairs, I stood momentarily outside the gym entrance. On the verge of a heart attack, I punched in my security code on the door. Dark, cold, and eerily quiet from the power being shut off, I apprehensively footed forward. From the first step in, water met my tennis shoes. Proceeding into the middle of the darkened room brought no relief. Flooded with over an inch of water across the 5,000 plus square feet, I was in complete shock.

I took several deep breaths and tried to envision solutions to the problem. After realizing this wasn't a nightmare, I started making multiple phone calls.

Two of my friends, Doug and Tom, arrived in minutes and the local disaster relief team was on its way. With headlamps glaring at the floor, we began using snow shovels to move water into floor drains. As strange as that probably sounds, we made pretty significant progress until the pros arrived. They had large vacuum hoses to remove excess water, fans for drying, and other tools to complete the mission.

With the power back on, more details of the damage were now visible. The ceiling, sheetrocked walls, lockers, and weight and cardio machines were all dripping with water. The carpeted areas were saturated and dozens of rubber mats were floating in the mess. I had just purchased a new treadmill and an elliptical trainer that were now coated in water. My biggest concerns were in my office, which housed the surveillance system, stereo, personal files, books, photos, and other irreplaceable memorabilia. Thankfully, most of it was only damp, but hundreds of members' workout cards were soaked. We were able to save most of them by separating and laying them against any remaining dry surfaces on the floor.

After a full day and night of removing carpet, pulling up rubber floor mats from under the heavy weight equipment, taking pictures off the walls, wiping down equipment, walls, and mirrors, it was time to go home.

Days later an insurance adjuster estimated my damage to be roughly $10,000. Thankfully this covered the emergency disaster team bill, flooring replacement, sheetrock repair/replacement, fitness equipment damage and multiple other miscellaneous items. Fortunately, out of the 16-plus-years that my 24/7 gym has been open, other than for moving to the space I now own, this was the only day we've been closed.

In the midst of all the chaos and frustration that day, I meditated on my breathing. I focused on breathing deep into my diaphragm instead of shallow into the lungs, like most of us normally do. My conscious breathing kept me from reacting to the flight-or-fight instinct, which would not have been productive under the circumstances. I kept repeating in my mind that "this too shall pass." It became my mantra to remain calm and effective through the ordeal.

"You have power over your mind - not outside events.
Realize this, and you will find strength."
~ Marcus Aurelius, Ancient Roman philosopher, emperor

Sunshine at all levels is harmful and should be avoided unless sunblock is applied.

Myth.

Natural sunlight triggers the production of vitamin D, the "sunshine vitamin." Vitamin D is a crucial ingredient for overall health and well-being. Vitamin D is actually an oil-soluble steroid hormone. It's formed when the skin is exposed to ultraviolet B (UVB) radiation from the sun. The proper amount of vitamin D lowers blood pressure, protects against inflammation, improves brain function, promotes weight loss, helps muscles, and may protect against certain cancers. Low vitamin D levels can increase heart disease, dementia, and prostate cancer. A recent study found that men who were deficient in vitamin D had more than double the normal risk of a heart attack. Vitamin D boosts your natural anti-inflammatory response, minimizing heart attacks.

Contrary to popular belief, we are meant to be in the sun. Once regarded as a divine power in some cultures, the sunlight has now been classified as a Class 1 carcinogen by the World Health Organization (WHO). Photobiologist Dr. Alexander Wunsch, CEO of Medical Light Consulting in Heidelberg, Germany wonders why. Once revered as a healing power, today sunlight is blamed for disease, and humans are urged to mostly shun this natural element.

Public and medical opinions of sunlight have changed drastically over time. In ancient times, sunlight was used for medical purposes like controlling germs and hardening bones. It was also used to treat tuberculosis and rickets.

According to Dr. Wunsch, "History demonstrates that natural, as well as artificial sunlight, can act as a major interventional tool to prevent and heal devastating diseases when used with diligence. Our ancestors had the skills, knowledge, and technologies to deal with the sunlight in all climate regions of our planet. Some of that cultural knowledge has vanished. Before the era of antibiotics, phototherapy (light therapy) was a state-of-the-art treatment in contemporary (alternative) medicine. The earliest records of light therapy go back five millennia to the ancient Egyptians. Modern era light therapy started in 1877, when Arthur Downes, MD, and Thomas Blunt, MA, two English scientists reported that exposure to light inhibited fungal growth in test tubes. When and where natural sunlight was not available, artificial sunlight was successfully used to fill the gap.

Sunlight can have a huge impact on depression, sleep quality, and seasonal affective disorder (SAD), a problem that affects about 10% of the U. S. population. Studies have shown that depressed people in general have low levels of vitamin D. Experts suggest 15-20 minutes in the sun a day is crucial for good health. Data shows that northern countries that have less sunlight have higher levels of heart disease than sunny southern countries. More heart attacks occur in the winter months when sunlight is scarce.

It's time to get outdoors, folks! Walk, bike, garden, ski, hike, golf, etc. Stop being afraid of the sun. We need its rays to survive and thrive. Just be mindful not to overexpose yourself and get burned.

Now the bad news. The other parts of the solar spectrum, like ultraviolet A (UVA) is harmful. In addition to coming directly from the sun, these rays can be emitted through windows and from indoor lighting. We need to be mindful not to be out in it too long without the proper sunscreen. The problem is there are many growing concerns around the side effects of cheap sunscreens. Minor irritations include redness, swelling, itching, aggravated acne, and eye irritation. An Environmental World Group (EWG) study of 783 sunscreens showed that 84% contained unsafe ingredients. Most, if not all, of which are now banned in Europe. Let's take a look at these six chemical ingredients that are absorbed into the skin, our body's second (behind fascia) largest organ!

Harmful ingredients found in common sunscreens are:

- **Oxybenzone** - enhances penetration of ingredients to get into the deeper layers of the skin. It can mimic, block, and alter hormones. The Center for Disease Control and Prevention (CDC) states that 97% of Americans have this chemical circulating in their bodies. This chemical can accumulate faster than our bodies can eliminate it.
- **Octinoxate** - a hormone disruptor that produces lots of free radicals that damage the skin and the cells, causing premature aging.
- **Retinyl Palmitate** (Vitamin A Palmitate) - Vitamin A is a good antioxidant, but when exposed to the sun it can promote spread of free radicals and the growth of cancerous tumors. A 2009 FDA study showed that this chemical can also damage DNA.

- **Homosalate** - helps the sunscreen to penetrate. Accumulates in the body faster than we can eliminate it, becoming toxic, and disrupting our hormones.
- **Octocrylene** - produces oxygen radicals that damage cells and cause mutations. It is also toxic to the environment.
- **Paraben preservatives** - can induce allergic reactions, hormone disruption, and reproductive toxicity. It may be a contributor to the rising incidence of breast cancer.

The obvious best forms of sun protection would be hats, clothing, and of course shade. However, there are numerous toxin-free natural sunscreens available. Those with zinc and titanium are the preferred choices. Here are some safe SPF natural sunscreens recommended by experts:

- Alba Botanica, Aubrey Organics, Badger, Block Island Organics, California Baby, Episencial Sunny Sunscreen, John Masters Organics

"A day without sunshine is like, you know, night."
~ Steve Martin, American actor, comedian, writer, producer, playwright, author, and musician

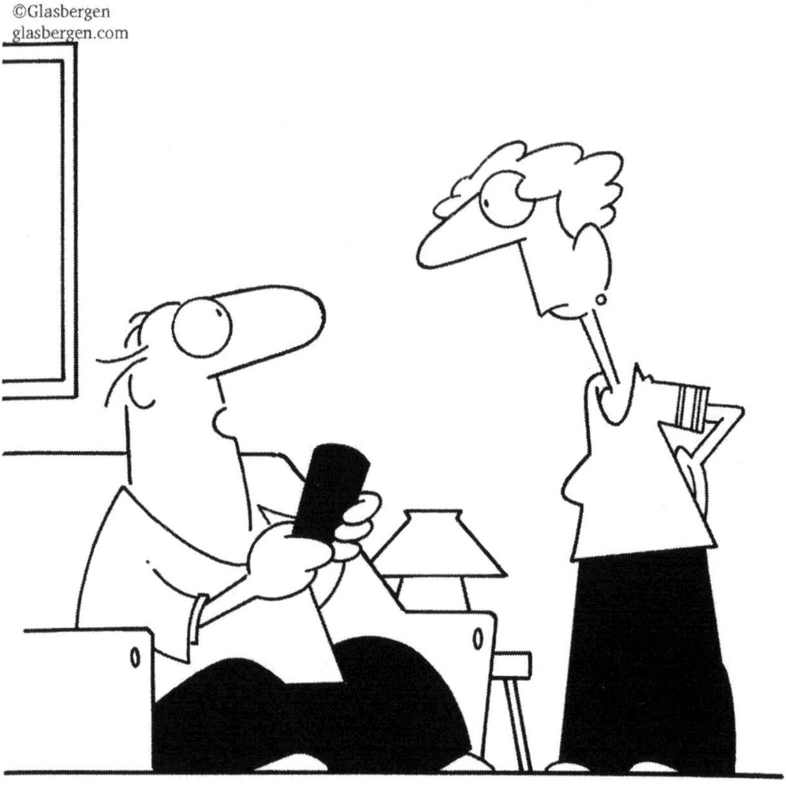

"My doctor says I need more fresh air and sunshine. I wonder if there's an app for that?"

Millions of Americans have parasites in them.

Fact.

According to the Centers for Disease Control, millions of Americans have parasites in their body. Found in food, water, and air, parasites are living organisms that pirate the nutrients of their host organism. This relationship is not symbiotic. You don't want parasites benefiting while depriving you of your nutrients. Not to be confused with beneficial microorganisms, these unwanted house guests can live throughout the body, but are found most commonly in the intestines.

For Americans, pork, shellfish, and contaminated water carry the highest risk of parasites. In developing nations, parasites are most commonly transmitted through contaminated water. Thousands of different types of parasites exist. If not identified, parasites can cause an infection in humans, which can lead to serious health problems, including seizures, pregnancy complications, blindness, heart failure, and even death. Parasites can usually be detected through a stool analysis or a blood test.

Once identified by the body, the immune system goes after them. The most common symptoms of parasites are gas, diarrhea, nausea, flu-like symptoms, joint pain, chronic fatigue, and more.

Parasites love sugar, so be sure to minimize this addictive anti-nutrient. If doing a cleanse, some people may see parasites in their stools, as they are being eliminated from the body.

There are many natural ways to help combat parasites:

- Onion
- Ginger
- Oregano
- Kimchee
- Raw garlic
- Sauerkraut
- Coconut oil
- Baking soda
- Apple cider vinegar
- Kombucha (low sugar variety)

Severe cases may need to be treated with anti-parasitic drugs or antibiotics. Seek a professional.

"Your diet is a bank account.
Good food choices are good investments."
~ Bethenny Frankel, American television personality, author, and entrepreneur

For the money, baking soda may be the healthiest, cheapest, and most versatile product on the market.

Fact.

Scientifically known as sodium bicarbonate, baking soda is naturally found in the mineral nahcolite, which exists in its pure form in the Green River Valley in Colorado. Baking soda's main benefit is that it neutralizes pH, keeping things from becoming overly acidic or overly alkaline.

For centuries, baking soda has been used as a raising agent when baking. However, this inexpensive and effective product has been used for numerous other things since ancient times.

The many health benefits of baking soda include:

- Helps digestive issues
- Reduces stomach pain
- Helps fight off diseases
- Neutralizes stomach acid
- Reduces bloating and gas
- Promotes kidney health
- Treats urinary tract infections
- Reduces the symptoms of gout
- Kills parasites, fungi, and mold
- Minimizes cough and sore throat
- Reduces muscle pain and fatigue
- Reduces the duration of cold and flu
- Minimizes lactic acid within the muscles

Baking soda is also a known exercise enhancer. It absorbs lactic acid that builds up in your muscles during intense workouts, delaying fatigue and enhancing athletic performance.

For indigestion, try the following:

Mix ½ teaspoon of baking soda dissolved in 4 ounces of water. Sip it slowly to avoid gas and diarrhea. Do not exceed 3 ½ teaspoons per day.

Most, if not all OTC (over-the-counter) antacids contain sodium bicarbonate.

Baking powder is different (not recommended) and only contains a little sodium bicarbonate.

Surprising uses for baking soda include:

- Natural deodorant; face exfoliator; hand softener; feet soother; itchy skin relief; splinter removal; bug bite soother; sunburn relief; hair cleanser; brush and comb cleaner; homemade toothpaste; teeth whitener and more.

Aluminum-free baking soda is your healthiest choice.

"For every drug that benefits a patient,
there is a natural substance that can achieve the same effect."
~ Pfeiffer's Law, Dr. Carl C. Pfeiffer, MD, PhD,
physician, biochemist

Epsom salt baths have astounding health benefits.

Fact.

Named after a bitter saline spring in Epsom, England, Epsom salt has been used for centuries to help everyone from gardeners who added it to their gardens for improving plant growth, to athletes with sore muscles who soaked in it. Unlike other naturally occurring salts, Epsom salt is formed from pure mineral compounds containing magnesium and sulfate. These minerals are absorbed through the epidermis, leaving the skin feeling soft and silky.

Bathing in Epsom salt has numerous benefits:

- **Eliminates toxins** using sulfates that trigger reverse osmosis
- **Stimulates nerve and muscle functions**
- **Reduces stress** by relaxing the muscles and the mind
- **Reduces pain and inflammation** (the root cause of most disease) and is a natural treatment for headaches (even migraines), as well as for bronchial asthma
- **Improves blood sugar levels**
- **Volumizes hair** by decreasing excess oil

Epsom Salts can be found at most drugstores and is very affordable.

"I'm really old-fashioned. An Epsom salt bath, that's genuinely better than any massage."
~ Emilia Clarke, English actress

Some essential oils are more effective than antibiotics in fighting superbugs.

Fact.

The alarming increase in superbugs in the last several years can primarily be attributed to antibiotic overuse. This overuse in people, livestock, and commercial products is leading to serious human illnesses, incurable infections, amputations, and even death. Too many antibiotics in beef, pork, poultry, medications, antibacterial hand soaps, and cleansers are resulting in a new breed of antibiotic-resistant bacteria.

The latest research shows that some new forms of bacteria are totally resistant to ALL forms of current antibiotics. In 2016, the United States dedicated $1.2 billion to fighting antibiotic resistance, and yet scientists are still losing this bacterial arms race.

Antibiotics kill most of the important microbiome (healthy bacteria) in our body, which help protect and preserve our immune system. In addition, healthy flora prevents the dangerous overgrowth of harmful bacteria, fungus, and viruses in our bodies. Beneficial bacteria improve mood and well-being, while reducing anxiety and depression. It can take up to a year to regrow a healthy population of gut bacteria after taking antibiotics.

Many essential oils combat antibiotic resistance and common harmful bacteria, as well as fungi and yeasts. Essential oils don't have the harmful side effects of antibiotics. These oils are applied to the skin or inhaled.

Hospitals are fighting a losing battle against man-made antibiotic-resistant bacteria. Scientists are now looking to herbal tonics such as essential oils to provide an answer. In 25 states, hospitals like Johns Hopkins Hospital in Baltimore; St Francis Hospital in Hartford, Connecticut; Wishard Memorial Hospital in Indianapolis, Indiana; Banner Health in Mesa, Arizona, are now using essential oils as alternatives to powerful and dangerous synthetic medical antibiotics.

Research from the Technological Educational Institute in Greece tested the antimicrobial activity of several essential plant oils. They found thyme to be the most effective essential oil and could almost completely eliminate bacteria within 60-minutes! Essential oils of thyme and cinnamon were found to be particularly effective at treating a range of Staph species. These strains are common inhabitants of the skin and some cause infection.

MARCoNS, a tricky strain of bacteria defined as a multiple antibiotic-resistant staph has been shown to be controlled with oregano oil and cinnamon oil. Oregano oil is a powerful natural antibiotic that's been used for centuries to treat wounds and infections, even staph infections. This amazing oil is antiviral, antioxidant, antifungal, antiparasitic, anti-inflammatory, and an anesthetic (pain reliever). Oregano oil contains carvacrol (liver cleanser and antioxidant) and thymol (helps strengthen the immune system and protect against toxins), two active ingredients that make it a powerful antibacterial. A 2001 Georgetown University Study found that oregano oil was just as effective as most antibiotics at treating athlete's foot, toenail fungus, sinus infections, and even pneumonia. Oregano oil is highly effective against Giardia, E Coli, Salmonella, Campylobacter and Staphylococcus. It is best not to use for more than two-weeks.

Another powerful natural antibiotic is cinnamon oil. Studies from Kansas State University and *The American Journal of Chinese Medicine* showed that cinnamon oil fights Staphylococcus, Aureus, E-coli, Pseudomonas, and Klebsiella. Cinnamon oil is an antioxidant, anti-parasitic, anti-inflammatory, digestive aid, blood sugar stabilizer, and blood circulation booster. It also relieves depression, increases the immune system, decreases cardiovascular diseases, and helps impotence. It is also used for dental bacteria, cavities, and root canals.

Tea Tree oil (Melaleuca), another promising natural antibiotic, has been shown to fight superbug MRSA (Methicillin-resistant Staphylococcus aureus) and speed up the healing process more effectively than medical antibiotic treatments. Australian Aborigines have used Tea Tree oil for thousands of years to treat colds, sore throats, skin infections, and insect bites. Tea Tree oil was also used as a commercial antiseptic in the early 20th Century. It was used extensively until penicillin was invented in 1928 by Alexander Fleming, Professor of Bacteriology at St. Mary's Hospital in London.

Rosemary oil also shows much promise with its antibacterial, antiviral, antioxidant, and anti-inflammatory properties. Research has shown that it can suppress the growth of 60 strains of E-coli in hospital patients. "Not only are essential oils a cheap and effective treatment option for antibiotic-resistant strains, but decreased use of antibiotics will help minimize the risk of new strains of antibiotic-resistant microorganisms emerging," said Technological

Education Institute of Ionian Islands Professor, Yiannis Samaras, in the Department of Food Technology.

Interestingly, some of these mentioned essential oils mixed with others, known as Thieves Oil, have been shown to have a powerful antibacterial effect as well. Legend has it that thieves back in the 15th Century robbed grave sites while avoiding contagions from the dead bodies. Their secret to avoiding sickness was a blend of clove, lemon, cinnamon, eucalyptus, and rosemary oils doused on a handkerchief that they placed over their mouths and noses. A 1996 lab test confirmed that a commercial Thieves Oil blend had a 90% effective rate against airborne bacteria. You may purchase a commercial blend or make your own.

The following is a vintage "Thieves Oil" recipe:

- 40 drops organic clove bud essential oil
- 35 drops organic lemon essential oil
- 20 drops organic cinnamon essential oil
- 15 drops organic eucalyptus oil
- 10 drops organic rosemary essential oil

I like to use a few drops of Thieves Oil (aka Protective Blend) mixed with water in a diffuser that sits in my office. The smell is fantastic!

Be mindful that regular grocery store varieties of essential oils won't do the trick. Therapeutic, medical grade oils must be used. All essential oil must be diluted in a carrier oil when applied topically. Do not take internally unless under the supervision of a healthcare practitioner.

"Frankincense is my second favorite f-word."
~ Unknown

Colors affect the human mind and body.

Fact.

"Most people are unaware of the profound effect color has on their behavior," states Kenneth Fehrman, co-author of the book, *Color: The Secret Influence,* which he wrote with this wife, Cherie Fehrman. Colors play a pivotal role in our lives and influence our activities and responses:

- **Red** - Stimulates the adrenal gland and neurons. Too much can cause stress and may also lead to anger and frustration. This color stimulates breathing and heartbeat. Wearing red clothes can make you appear heavier. Red also increases the appetite - no wonder the fast food industry uses this color regularly. The color red also helps with focusing and memory.
- **Pink** - Found to reduce anger and anxiety. Evokes romance, love, and friendship.
- **Orange** - A mood enhancer, it stimulates mental abilities. It also increases the appetite. Associated with joy, enthusiasm, creativity, fascination, and determination.
- **Yellow** - Releases serotonin which causes a happy mood. However, too much gives the brain and the nervous system fatigue. Speeds up the metabolism and is a common food color. Associated with intellect, energy, comfort, liveliness, and optimism.
- **Green** - Soothing on the eyes. Relaxes the body and relieves stress. Think nature! Yoga studios are generally painted some shade of green. Green

improves vision. This ubiquitous natural color has a healing and hygienic effect. Studies show that consumers spend more time in shops painted green.

- **Blue** - Enhances creativity. Producing calming chemicals in the brain, blue has a soothing effect on the human mind. Too much exposure, however, may cause depression. Denotes loyalty. Materials blue in color appear to be lighter in weight. Blue is a non-food color and gives off a toxic effect to edibles.
- **Purple** - Symbolizes royalty, luxury, sophistication. Develops deep thinking and spirituality. Intensifies sexual activity.
- **Black** - Signifies authority and power. Represents knowledge and intelligence. Associated with "style" in the fashion industry and is popular because it makes people look thinner. It is the most aggressive color. Research shows that hockey teams wearing black are penalized more for fouls.
- **White** - Most neutral color. Symbolizes cleanliness and innocence. Associated with sophistication in the clothing industry. Studies show that people having hand tremors don't shake as much in white rooms, proving its calming effect.

"The soul becomes dyed with the color of its thoughts."
~ Marcus Aurelius, Roman emperor

The color of a food indicates the healing properties within that food.

Fact.

Colors can tell a lot about the food you eat. Consider the following:

Red Foods

- Foods that are red speed up your circulation by heating your body. They contain lycopene, a powerful antioxidant that prevents cancer development and inflammation in the arteries. Mix with fat to increase bioavailability. Red foods include beets, cherries, chilies, cranberries, radishes, raspberries, red apples, red cabbage, red grapes, red peppers, rhubarb, strawberries, tomatoes, and watermelons.

Orange Foods

- Orange foods serve as an antispasmodic aid for pain and cramps. They help to strengthen the lungs in polluted environments and increase vitality and mental clarity. High in beta carotene, they help stabilize the immune system. Orange foods include apricots, butternut squash, cantaloupes, carrots, mangoes, oranges, papayas, pumpkin, and yams.

Yellow Foods

- The following motor-stimulants get you going faster in the morning by strengthening nerves and helping with digestion and constipation. Yellow foods include bananas, grapefruits, lemons, mangos, pineapples, yellow apples, yellow peaches, yellow peppers, and yellow squash.

Green Foods

- Green foods are a blood cleanser, bactericide, natural tranquilizer, and nutrifier. Green foods include avocados, broccoli, cucumber, green leafy veggies, green peppers, sea veggies, sprouts, and wheatgrass.

Blue/Purple Foods

- High in anthocyanins, the following fruits and vegetables belong to a phytochemical group that are known for helping to prevent cancer: blackberries, blueberries, eggplant, plums, red cabbage, and red grapes.

White Foods

- These power foods contain allicins, which combat viral and bacterial infections, support heart health, and help fight cancer. White foods include cauliflower, garlic, leeks, onions, and scallions.

"Let food be thy medicine and medicine be thy food."

~ Hippocrates, Father of Medicine, Greek physician

Suggested Resources

Books to read:

- *3 Worst Medications You're Probably Taking; Over-The-Counter Natural Cures; Hidden Truth About Cholesterol Lowering Drugs; Health Myths Exposed,* Shane Ellison, MS
- *The Metabolic Approach to Cancer,* Dr. Nasha Winters, ND, LAC, FABNO, Jess Higgins Kelly, MNT
- *Sugar Nation: The Hidden Truth Behind America's Deadliest Habit and the Simple Way to Beat It,* Jeff O'Connell
- *Good Calories, Bad Calories; The Case Against Sugar, Why We Get Fat: And What To Do About It,* Gary Taubes
- *Spark: The Revolutionary New Science of Exercise and the Brain,* John J. Ratey, MD
- *The Telomere Effect, The New Science of Living Younger,* Elizabeth Blackburn, PhD, and Elissa Epel, PhD
- *Deep Nutrition: Why Your Genes Need Traditional Food,* Catherine Shanahan, MD
- *Advances in Functional Training,* Mike Boyle
- *Prescription for Nutritional Healing,* James Balch, MD, and Phyllis Balch, CNC
- *The New Rules of Lifting for Women: Lift Like a Man, Look Like a Goddess,* Lou Schuler and Alwyn Cosgrove

- *Ultimate Back Fitness and Performance,* Stuart McGill, PhD
- *Facts and Fallacies of Fitness,* Dr. Mel Siff

Movies to watch:

- The Magic Pill, 2018
- Fed Up, 2014
- Hungry for Change, 2012
- Farmageddon, 2011
- Food, Inc., 2009
- Food Matters, 2008
- Super Size Me, 2004

Author's Summary

Sufficient exercise, proper nutrition, and adequate sleep provide a heightened sense of self. Being healthy, physically and mentally, enhances all aspects of life. With better strength, stamina, balance, flexibility, and mobility, the body is more capable of performing all the outdoor and indoor activities that we enjoy. Exercise also enhances our clarity of mind. With increased blood flow and the release of endorphins in the brain, our mood is elevated and our senses heightened.

The secret to achieving your fitness and nutrition goals is about lifestyle choices, not life-changing transformations. Start with some small changes and watch what happens. A positive mental attitude, a consistent exercise routine, a healthy eating plan, all with enough sleep, are what will carry you to wherever it is that you want to go.

It is time to set realistic goals with specific times and dates and be consistent by sticking to that schedule. This will create new daily habits that you will be proud of forever.

More than just survive, it's time to thrive! So, open your wellness toolbox to optimize your health.

To a vibrant life,
Don

Author's Credentials

- National Academy of Sports Medicine (N.A.S.M.) Personal Fitness Trainer
- American Council on Exercise (A.C.E.) Lifestyle & Weight Management Consultant
- Certified TRX Group Fitness Instructor
- Founder/Owner of Fitness Solutions 24/7 gym since 2002
- Gym designer (1993, 1995, 2002, 2008)
- Colorado Natural Bodybuilding Championships competitor, 3rd place - 2006, 5th place – 1996
- Fitness Business Consultant

References

Section One

Physical activity, not drugs, is our best defense against everything from mood disorders to Alzheimer's disease to ADHD to addiction. Fact. p. 19

Godman, H., "Regular Exercise Changes the Brain to Improve Memory, Thinking Skills," healthharvard.edu, 4/5/18

Ratey, J., MD, *Spark, The Revolutionary New Science of Exercise and the Brain,* 2008

"Stopping Brain Drain," *What Doctors Don't Tell You,* January 2007

Kids shouldn't start lifting weights until they're at least 12 years old. Myth. p. 27

Doheny, K., "Is Weight Training Safe for Kids?" webmd.com, n.d.

"Kids Fitness Programs: Should They Really Lift Weights?" iyca.org, 2009

"Myth: Weightlifting Makes Kids Short," positionusa.com, 7/23/17

Siff, M., *Facts and Fallacies of Fitness,* 1995

Crunches and sit-ups isolate the abdominal muscles, and give you the best chance of developing a lean midsection and six pack. Myth. p. 30

Gottschall, J., Mills, J., Hastings, B., Penn State University, Les Mills International, "Optimal Core Training for

Functional Gains and Peak Performance: CWWORX," n.d.
Lippincott, Williams, and Wilkins, *ACSM's Guidelines for Exercise Testing and Prescription*, 2005
"Strength Training: Work the Floor of Your Core," healthiq.com, 6/5/18

Cardiovascular exercise is the best way to lose body fat. Myth. p. 33

Baye, D., "Fat Loss Myths Part 2: Cardio Is Necessary For Fat Loss," baye.com, 7/01/08
Fetters, A., "What's Best for Weight Loss: Cardio or Strength Training?" womanshealthmag.com, 11/22/13
Robertson, M., "4 Reasons to Choose Strength Training Over Cardio," livestrong.com, 5/16/17

Women and men should do the same exercises when it comes to weight training. Fact. p. 36

Richardson, K., "Should Women Train & Lift Weights Like Men?" naturallyintense.net, 1/20/17
Schuler, L., Forsythe, C., M.S., Cosgrove, A., *The New Rules of Lifting For Women*, 2007
Siff, M. Dr., *Facts and Fallacies of Fitness*, 2003
White, C., "Should Men and Women Train Differently?" abc.net.au, 5/31/17

Lifting free weights is safer and more effective than using weight machines. Fact. p. 38

Hall, B., "Game Changer: Should You Be Using Machines or Free Weights?" stack.com, 1/12/15
Schuler, L., Cosgrove, A., *The New Rules of Lifting Supercharged Deluxe*, 2012
"The Pros and Cons of Free Weights versus Resistance Machines," fitness.mercola.com, 12/12/14

High-intensity interval training (HIIT) has more benefits than traditional cardio. Fact. p. 43

Colino, S., "The Surprising Perks of High-Intensity Interval Training," health.usnews.com, 5/10/17

Kravitz, L., PhD, *HIIT Your Limit: High-Intensity Interval Training for Fat Loss, Cardio, and Full Body Health,* 10/9/18

Tinsley, G., PhD., "7 Benefits of High Intensity Interval Training," healthline.com, 6/2/17

Functional training is fun, fast, and purposeful. Fact. p. 46

Boyle, M., New Functional Training for Sports, 2016

Morjaria, C., "What is Functional Training," breakingmuscle.com, n.d

Richardson, G., "7 Benefits of Functional Training," linkedin.com, 2/23/15

Sweating is a sign of being out of shape. Myth. p. 51

Borrelli, L., "Sweat It Out! 5 Surprising Benefits Of Sweating That Actually Don't Stink," medicaldaily.com, 11/7/14

Kumar, P., "9 Myths About Sweat," boldsky.com, 9/23/15

"5 Myths and 1 Truth About Summer Sweat," sweathelp.org, n.d.

"More Sweat = More Calories Burned," orthology.com, 2/28/17

"Myths and Facts about Excessive Sweating," skincareguide.com, n.d.

It is not possible to be fat and fit. Myth. p. 53

Chodosh, S., "Fat but Fit is Absolutely Possible, popsci.com, 5/29/17

Rosen, P., "Can You Be Fat But Fit?" fitnessmagazine.com, June 2013

BMI (body mass index) is a poor way to determine one's state of health. Fact. p. 55

Cespedes, A., "Problems With BMI," livestrong.com, July 2017

Devlin, K., "Top 10 Reasons Why The BMI Is Bogus," nprradio.com, 7/4/09

Gupta, Dr. S., "What's Wrong With BMI?" EverydayHealth.com, 4/29/13

Full-body weight training workouts are better than split routines (one or two body parts worked per day) for strength and conditioning. Fact. p. 57

Clark, S., "The Top 10 Reasons To Use Full Body Workouts," bodybuilding.com, 4/1/10

Rogers et al, "The Effect of Supplemental Isolated Weight-Training Exercises on Upper-Arm Size and Upper-Body Strength," Human Performance Laboratory, Ball State University, Muncie, IN. NSCA Conference Abstract, 2000

Smith, B., "Ask Men's Fitness: Is it Better to Do Full-body Workouts or Body-part Focused Routines?" mensjournal.com, n.d.

Waterbury, C., "Total Body Training: The 3-Day-Per-Week, Full Body Workout Plan," tnation.com, 10/11/04

Deadlifts are just as effective as bicep curls and tricep extensions for arm strength and size. Fact. p. 60

Boyle, M., "Are You Afraid of Deadlifts?" strengthcoach.com, n.d.

Robson, D., "Deadlifts: The King of Mass-Builders," bodybuilding.com, 8/28/17

"The Effect of Supplemental Isolated Weight Training Exercises on Upper Arm Size and Upper Body Strength"

Human Performance Laboratory, Ball State University, Muncie, Indiana, NSCA Conference Abstract, 2000

Squats are complicated and dangerous, causing knee and back problems. Myth. p. 62

Clark, D., Lambert, M., Hunter, A., "Muscle Activation in the Loaded Free Barbell Squat: A Brief Review," J Strength Cond. Res 26(4): 1169-1178, 2012
DuVall, J., M.S., C.P.T., "Get Stronger: 7 Reasons You Should Never Neglect Squats," mensfitness.com, n.d.
"How to Do Squats: 8 Reasons to Do Squat Exercises," fitness.mercola.com, 5/25/12
Reynolds, G., "Brawn and Brains," nytimes.com, 11/18/15

Running causes knee problems and arthritis. Myth. p. 67

Cox, L., "5 Experts Answer: Is Running Bad for Your Knees?" livescience.com, 4/6/12
Hutchinson, A., "Here's More Evidence That Running Doesn't Ruin Your Knees," runnersworld.com, 2/6/17
Reynolds, G., Why Runners Don't Get Knee Arthritis," well.blogs.nytimes.com, 9/25/13

After age 60, you cannot gain muscle mass or strength. Myth. p. 69

Neighmond, P., "Seniors Can Still Bulk Up On Muscle By Pressing Iron," npr.com, 2/21/11
Reynolds, G., "Can You Regain Muscle Mass After Age 60?" newyorktimes.com, 12/2/16
"Sarcopenia: 10 Keys to Keep Your Muscle Mass," draxe.com, n.d.

We are all pre-programmed to live a certain number of years. Our genetics determine this. Exercise and nutrition have very little to do with it. Myth. p. 72

Joseph, A., Bronshtein, N., "Even With Medical Advances, Humans May Not Live Past 130" pbs.org, 10/6/16

Woollaston, V. "We'll Soon All Live To 120 Years Old - But This Is Probably the Absolute Limit," dailymail.co.uk, 10/22/14

Unless you are a competitive athlete, setting fitness/nutrition goals is basically a waste of time. Myth. p. 74

Clear, J., "Goal Setting: A Scientific Guide to Setting and Achieving Goals," jamesclear.com, n.d.

Holbrook, S., "5 Ways to Set Effective Goals and Beat Burnout," health.usnews.com, 1/13/14

Traugott, J., "Achieving Your Goals: An Evidence-based Approach," msue.anr.msu.edu, 8/26/14

Visualization techniques and practices can have a profound effect on achieving your goals. Fact. p. 77

Kehoe, J., "Visualizations," learnmindpower.com, n.d.

LeVan, A., "Seeing is Believing: The Power of Visualization," psychologytoday.com, 12/3/09

Williams, A., "8 Successful People Who Use The Power Of Visualization," mindbodygreen.com, 7/8/15

There are no proven ways for getting motivated to exercise. Myth. p. 82

Lawler, M., "Move It! Scientifically Proven Ways to Get Motivated," fitnessmagazine.com, n.d.

Macha, A., "6 Science-Based Secrets to Staying Motivated at the Gym," nbcnews.com, 1/03/18

Smith-Janssen, K., "10 Weird Ways to Make Yourself Workout-Even When You Really Don't Want To," prevention.com, n.d.

Keeping a journal for your exercise and nutrition records can double a person's weight loss. Fact. p. 84

Connery, R., "5 Reasons Why You Should Keep a Fitness Journal," active.com, n.d.
"Training Diary/Log/Journal," healthiq.com, March 2018

The best exercises for developing the calf muscles don't involve typical weight training exercises. Fact. p. 87

Haley, A., "Why Calf Raises Are a Waste of Time," stack.com, 7/18/14
Siff, M., Dr., *Facts and Fallacies of Fitness*, 2003
Waterbury, C., M.S., "Tip: Discover the Single-Best Calf Exercise," tnation.com, 5/13/16

Jumping rope is far more effective than jogging for improving cardiovascular efficiency. Fact. p. 91

Baker, J. A., "Comparison of Rope Skipping and Jogging as Methods of Improving Cardiovascular Efficiency of College Men," tandfonline.com, 3/17/13
Carerra, M & Vani, N., "The Best Exercise for Weight Loss," weightloss.com.au, 9/22/06
Cook, G., MSPT, OCS, CSCS, "Self-limiting Exercise: Jumping Rope," *Athletic Body in Balance*, pp 125-129, performance.nd.edu, 2003
Heid, M., "Why Jumping Rope is a Shockingly Good Workout," timeinc.net, 7/14/17
Robson, D., "Which Cardio Methods Melt Fat The Fastest," bodybuilding.com, 12/15/17

Rebounding (jumping on a mini-trampoline) is as beneficial as jogging. Fact. p. 94

Bhattacharya, E., McCutcheon, E.P., Shvartz, E., Greenleaf, J.E., "Body Acceleration Distribution and O2 Uptake in Humans During Running and Jumping," physiology.org, 1980

Carter, A., "Rebounding: Science Behind the 7 Major Health Benefits of Rebound Exercise," cancertutor.com, 12/11/17

"Spring Into Health With a Rebounding Workout," healthiq.com, 3/22/18

"Why Rebounding is So Beneficial," HealingDaily.com, 2009

Whole Body Vibration is a useless method of exercise. Myth. p. 96

"A Brief History of Accelerated Vibration Training," 3gcardio.com, n.d.

Bosco, C., et al., "Hormonal Responses to Whole-body Vibration in Men," European Journal of Applied Physiology, 81:449-454, 2000

Mercola, J., ND, "The Many Health Benefits of Whole Body Vibrational Training," fitnessmercola.com, 4/7/17

Rittweger, J., et al., "Treatment of Chronic Lower Back Pain with Lumbar Extension and Whole Body Vibration Exercise," 2002

"Whole Body Vibration May be as Effective as Regular Exercise," endocrine.org, 3/15/17

Jack LaLanne (1914-2011) was the greatest pioneer in the world of fitness. Fact. p. 100

Clear, J., "Learning From a Superhuman: The Incredible Fitness and Success of Jack LaLanne," huffpost.com, 7/6/13

Robbin, J., "Jack LaLanne Dies: Who the Fitness Guru Really Was," huffpost.com, 5/25/11

Goldstein, R. "Jack LaLanne, Founder of Modern Fitness Movement, Dies at 96," mobile.nytimes.com, 1/23/11

No trainer in history has brought more to bodybuilding than Vince Gironda (1917- 1997). Fact. p.103

Gironda, V., Unleashing the Wild Physique, 1984
Heimbuch, K., "Vince Gironda's 8x8 Workout," oldschooltrainer.com, 7/28/16
Thibaudeau, C., "The Gironda System," tnation.com, 6/08/06

The psoas may be the most important muscle in the body. Fact. p. 108

Axe, J., DNM, DC, CNS, "A Weak Psoas Muscle Could Be The Cause of that Back Pain," draxe.com, 10/2/16
"Get to Know Your Psoas Muscles," berkeleywellness.com, 2/26/18
Northrup, C., MD, "Why Your Psoas Muscle Is The Most Vital Muscle In Your Body," drnorthrup.com, 6/5/18

Scientists have found a new organ called fascia; it could be the largest in your body. Fact. p. 111

Howard, J., "Newfound Organ Could Be the Biggest In Your Body," cnn.com, 3/31/18
"Interstitium: 'New' Organ Found in Human Body," sci-news.com, 3/28/18
Thomas, B., "The Top 5 Ways Fascia Matters To Athletes," breakingmuscle.com, n.d.

Static stretching is an outdated methodology that should not be used. Myth. p. 116

Cressey, E., "Coaching Cues to Make Your Strength and Conditioning Programs More Effective-Installment 6," ericcressey.com, n.d.

Page, P., PT, PhD, ATC, CSCS, FACSM, "Current Concepts in Muscle Stretching for Exercise and Rehabilitation," ncbi.nlm.nih.gov, 2012

"The Effects of Static Stretching and Warm-up Exercise on Hamstring Length over 24 Hours," *Journal of Orthopedics and Sports Therapy*, Volume 33, Number 12, P 727-733, December 2003

Couples who train together tend to stay together. Fact. p. 120

DiDonato, E., Ph.D., "5 Reasons Why Couples Who Sweat Together, Stay Together," psychologytoday.com, 1/10/14

"The Perfect Workout Partner: Why Couples Who Sweat Together Stay Together," huffpost.com, 2/10/13

Whistance, B., "Couples That Train Together, Remain Together," get-a-wingman.com, n.d.

13-minute weight training workouts are sufficient for muscular strength and endurance. Fact. p. 122

Blewett, D., "20-Minute Muscle: Better Gains Through Shorter Workouts," bodybuilding.com, 1/13/16

Eastman, H., NSCA, CPT, "Achieve the Same Gains with Shorter Workouts," bodybuilding.com, 7/27/17

MacDonald, F., "Short Weight-Lifting Sessions Can Improve Your Memory," sciencealert.com, 10/6/14

Reynolds, G., "In a Hurry? Try Express Weight Training," nytimes.com, 9/12/18

Section Two

No references

Section Three

Weight gain and weight loss is all about calories in and calories out. Myth. p. 161

Kollias, H., "Weight Loss and Hunger Hormones: Why Willpower May Not Be Your Problem," precisionnutrition.com, n.d.
Marion, J., "The Biggest Nutrition Myth Ever," nutritionwatchdog.com, 12/22/15
Sumithran, P., Prendergast, L., Delbridge, E., Purcell, K., Shulkes, A., Kriketos, A., Proietto, J., "Long Term Persistence of Hormonal Adaptations to Weight Loss," N Engl J Med;365(17):1597-604, 10/27/11
Teta, J., Dr., "Want to Lose Fat? Count Your Hormones, Not Your Calories," huffingtonpost.com, 1/8/13

If you have high cholesterol, you have heart disease. Myth. p. 164

Helmer, J., "Everything You Thought You Knew About Cholesterol Is Wrong," aarp.com, 2/20/15
Mercola, J., ND, "Cholesterol Myths You Need to Stop Believing," articles.mercola.com, 4/20/16
Perlmutter, D., MD, *Grain Brain*, 2013

Consuming saturated fat is healthy. Fact. p. 168

Alakbarli, F., Dr., "Nutrition for Longevity," *Azerbaijan International*, pages 20-23, Autumn 2000
"Association of Fats and Carbohydrates Intake with Cardiovascular Disease and Mortality in 18 Countries from

Five Continents (PURE): a Prospective Cohort Study," lancet.com, 8/29/17

Enig, M., Ph.D., Expert in Lipid Biochemistry, "The Truth About Saturated Fats," n.d.

Gunnars, K., BSc, "Top 8 Reasons Not to Fear Saturated Fats," 2/25/13

"Reducing Total Fat Intake May Have Small Effects or Risk of Breast Cancer, No Effects or Risk of Colon Cancer, Heart Disease or Stroke," nih.gov, 2/07/06

All carbohydrates are absorbed quickly and convert into fat. Myth. p. 172

Geary, M., CNS, "Truth about Carbs," truthaboutcarbs.com, n.d.

"Managing Your Blood Sugar," newhealthadvisor.com, 12/3/15

Zaine, C., "All Carbs Are Not Created Equal," bodybuilding.com, 3/30/15

"Carb cycling" is one of the best ways to burn body fat. Fact. p. 174

Hadsall, S., *4 Cycle Fat Loss*, 2012

McDonald, L., *The Ultimate Diet 2.0*, 2003

Reynolds, B., Jade, N., *Sliced*, 1991

Robb, J., *The Fat Burning Diet*, 2004

Sugar is responsible for increases in heart disease, cancer, diabetes, high blood pressure, obesity and the weakening of our immune system. Fact. p. 180

Brueck, H., "Sugar," businessinsider.com, 11/21/17

Hyman, M., Dr., *The Blood Sugar Solution 10-day Detox Diet*, 2014

Skerrett, P., "Huge New Study Casts Doubt on Conventional Wisdom about Fat and Carbs," statnews.com, 8/29/17

"Sugar and Your Immune System," alternativehealthatlanta.com, 2017

Raw honey has multiple health benefits that have been known about for thousands of years. Fact. p. 186

"5 Things You Didn't Know About Honey," mercola.com, 10/20/14

LaMotte, S., "The Proven Health Benefits of Honey," m.cnn.com, 3/9/18

"The Many Health Benefits of Raw Honey," draxe.com, n.d.

Blackstrap molasses is just another camouflaged sugar. Myth. p. 189

"Blackstrap Molasses Combats Stress & Promotes Healthy Skin," draxe.com, n.d.

McDonnell, K., RD, "Everything You Need to Know About Molasses," medicalnewstoday.com, 7/31/17

Wholesome Sweeteners Organic Molasses label

A gluten-free diet will make you lose weight. Myth. p. 194

Barnes, Z., "5 Myths About Going Gluten-Free," womenshealth.com, 8/6/14

Corleone, J., RDN, LD, "Gluten Intolerance & Sourdough Bread," livestrong.com, 10/3/17

Geary, M., CNS, CPT, Ebeling, C., "3 Reasons THIS Kind of Bread is Healthier to Eat," thenutritionwatchdog.com, n.d

Sass, C., "6 Myths about Gluten-free Diets You Shouldn't Believe," health.com, 9/13/17

Sutherlin, F., "Don't Be Fooled by No. 1 Myth," *Durango Herald*, Food and Nutrition, 8/22/18

Fruit juice is not a healthy substitute for soda. Fact. p. 199

Cheng, E., Fiechtner, L., Carroll, A., "Seriously, Juice is Not Healthy," nytimes.com, 7/8/18

Ducharme, J., "The Case Against Juice Is Stronger Than Ever," timeinc.com, 1/25/18

Gunnars, C., BSc, "Fruit Juice Is Just as Unhealthy as a Sugary Drink," healthline.com, 6/4/17

Sports/energy drinks are healthy. Myth. p. 201

Dossantos, N., "The 13 Most Dangerous Energy Drinks," msn.com, 1/19/17

Fagan, J., PhD, Burgdorfer, L., Ogwang, S., Krajewski, A., "The Unseen Dangers of Sports and Energy Drinks," rucore.libraries.rutgers.edu, Summer, 2011

Olsen, N., RD, LD, ACSM EP-C, Schaefer, A., "Is Gatorade Bad for You," healthline.com, 7/10/17

Swanson, A., "Best and Worst Electrolyte Drinks," thehealthbeat.com, 7/21/13

"Top 14 Energy Drink Dangers," caffeineinformer.com, 3/5/18

Artificial sweeteners are a safe alternative to natural sweeteners. Myth. p. 205

Freidson, M., "The Soda Belly Diet," *Men's Health*, pp 117-121, July/August 2018

Mercola, J., ND, "Top 10 Destructive Nutrition Lies Ever Told," articles.mercola.com, 7/16/14

Mercola, J., ND, "What Is Luo Han Guo Good For?" mercola.com, 8/20/18

Strawbridge, H., "Artificial Sweeteners: Sugar-Free, But At What Cost?" healthharvard.edu, 1/8/18

"The 5 Worst Artificial Sweeteners," draxe.com, 2014

Drinking water can increase energy, boost your metabolism, decrease constipation, and may reduce cancer. Fact. p. 208

Boschmann, M., Steiniger, J., Hille, U., Tank, J., Adams, F., Sharma, A., Klaus, S., Luft, F., Jordan, J., "Water-Induced Thermogenesis," *Journal of Clinical Endocrinology and Metabolism*, Volume 88, Issue 12, pages 6015-6019, 12/01/03

David, Y.B., Gesundheit, B., Urkin, J., Kapelushnik, J., "Water Intake and Cancer Prevention," *Journal of Clinical Oncology*, ascopubs.org, 1/15/04

Sutherlin, F., RD, "Drink Water to Boost Your Brain Function," Healing Nutrition, *The Durango Herald*, 5/30/18

Yerba Mate may be the healthiest drink on the planet. Fact. p. 211

Axe, J., Dr., "Yerba Mate: Healthier than Green Tea & a Cancer Killer?" draxe, 1/21/16

"11 Impressive Benefits of Yerba Mate," organicfacts.net, 4/9/18

Petre, A., MS, RD, "8 Health Benefits of Yerba Mate (Backed by Science)," healthline.com, 7/3/16

Drinking coffee can potentially decrease the risk of numerous diseases and help you increase your metabolism. Fact. p. 215

Doherty, M. and Smith, P.M, "Effects of Caffeine on Exercise Testing: A Meta-analysis," *International Journal of Sports Nutrition, Exercise and Metabolism*, (6):626-46, 12/14/04

Gunnars, K., BSc, "Can Coffee Increase Your Metabolism and Help You Burn Fat?" healthline.com, 5/4/18

Presented at SLEEP 2016, the 30th Anniversary Meeting of the Associated Professional Sleep Societies, 6/13/16

"6 Reasons to Drink Coffee Before Your Workout," Mercola.com, 7/11/14

Chocolate should only be consumed on rare occasions. Myth. p. 218

Gunnars, K., BSc, "7 Proven Health Benefits of Dark Chocolate," healthline.com, 5/30/17

Hubbard, B., "Chocolate Every Day Keeps You Mentally Sharp in Every Way," wddty.com, 7/7/17

Mercola, J., ND, "The Amazing Health Benefits of Dark Chocolate," mercola.com, 2/8/16

Feed a cold, starve a fever. Myth. p. 222

DerSarkissian, C., "Starve a Cold, Feed a Fever?" webmd.com, 1/25/17

Fischetti, M, Senior Editor, "Fact or Fiction?: Feed a Cold, Starve a Fever?" scientificamerican.com, 1/3/14

O'Connor, A., "The Claim: Starve a Cold, Feed a Fever," mobilenytimes.com, 2/13/07

Kelp is a supergreen. Fact. p. 224

Jockers, D., DC, MS, CSCS., "6 Major Health Benefits of Sea Kelp," drjockers.com, n.d.

"Never Underestimate the Power of Kelp on Your Brain," getmomental.com, 11/28/17

Pletcher, P., MS, RD, LD, CDE, Buettner, K., "Kelp Benefits: A Health Booster from the Sea," healthline.com, 7/30/15

"The Anti-Inflammatory, Iodine-Rich Power of Kelp," draxe.com, 8/25/16

Protein is an overrated nutrient that should be consumed minimally. Myth. p. 226

Fetters, A., "How Much Protein Do You Really Need?" health.usnews.com, 12/11/15

Patz, A., "This Is How Much Protein You Really Need to Eat in a Day," health.com, 3/6/17

Pendick, D., "How Much Protein Do You Need Every Day?" 1/8/18

Eggs labeled "cage-free" are a scam. Fact. p. 229

Geary, M., CNS, "Why Cage-Free Eggs are a Scam (Eat These Instead)," thenutritionwatchdog.com, n.d.

Pope, S., "Why Organic Eggs from the Store are a Scam," thehealthyhomeeconomist.com, 8/30/18

The most powerful superfood is a plant. Myth. p. 231

Marshall, M., How to Build a Classic Physique, 2011

Seymour, T., "Are Organ Meats Good for You?" Benefits and Risks," medicalnewstoday.com, 9/3/17

Rowles, A., RD, "Why Liver Is a Nutrient-Dense Superfood," healthline.com, 6/7/17

Testosterone is a hormone that is boosted naturally with food. Fact. p. 233

Bailey, R., "10 of the Best Testosterone Boosting Foods," menshealth.co.uk, 1/31/18

Kadey, M., MS, RD, "The 6 Best Testosterone-Boosting Foods!" bodybuilding.com, 10/26/17

Mercola, J., ND, "7 Testosterone Boosting Foods," fitness.mercola.com, 4/8/16

All salt is basically the same, causes high blood pressure and should be minimized. Myth. p. 236

Aragon, A., M.S., "The Truth Behind 5 Food Myths," menshealth.com, 4/20/15

"Pink Himalayan Salt Benefits that Make It Superior to Table Salt," draxe.com, 1/1/17

Sheridan, M., "The Truth About Salt & Hypertension (High Blood Pressure), m.huffpost.com, 4/25/17

Known as the gold standard, bananas are nature's best source of potassium. Myth. p. 240

Lanham-New, S., Lambert, H., Frassetto, L., "Potassium - Advances in Nutrition," academic.oup.com, 11/6/12

"Power of Potassium," mercola.com, 4/25/16

Reynolds, B., Jade N., *Sliced,* 1991

"10 Advantages of Maintaining Healthy Potassium Levels," healthfacty.com, 4/24/18

It's only slightly more expensive to eat healthy food than it is to eat junk food. Fact. p. 242

Bittman, M., "Is Junk Food Really Cheaper?" newyorktimes.com, 9/24/11

Foods in a Low-Income Model," Family Medicine, stfm.org, April 2010

McDermott, A., ENS, MC, USN, Stephens, M., MD, CAPT, MC, USN, "Cost of Eating: Whole Foods Versus Convenience," nytimes.com, 1/07/16

Polis, C., "Eating Healthy Versus Unhealthy Will Cost You $550 More Per Year, Study Reveals," huffpost.com, 1/23/14

Soy is one of the healthiest foods on earth. Myth. p. 245

"Effects of Antenatal Exposure to Phytoestrogens on Human Male Reproductive and Urogenital Development," westonaprice.org, 11/16/05

Gunnars, K., BSc, "Is Soy Bad For You, or Good? The Shocking Truth," healthline.com, 9/22/13

"Soy: Eating This 'Health' Food? It Could Be Slowly and Silently Killing You," mercola.com, 12/4/10

Tarantino, O., "14 Things That Happen To Your Body When You Eat Soy," eatthis.com, 4/19/16

"The Little Known Soy-Gluten Connection," westonaprice.org, 6/28/10

More than ninety percent of cancer is the result of a poor diet and an unhealthy lifestyle. Fact. p. 249

Jockers, D., DC, MS, CSCS, "12 Ways to Prepare for a Detox Cleanse," thetruthaboutcancer.com, January 2017

Sircus, M., AC, OMD, DM(P), "Cancer, Sulfur, Garlic & Glutathione," drsircus.com, 6/25/2012

Turner, K., PhD, *Radical Remission,* NY Times bestseller, 2014

Winters, N., Dr., ND, Kelley, J.H., MNT, The *Metabolic Approach to Cancer,* 2017

Fresh fruits and vegetables are always more nutritious than frozen varieties. Myth. p. 257

Brown, M.J., "Vegetables-Which Are Healthier?" healthline.com, 6/15/17

"Foods-Fresh vs. Frozen or Canned," medlineplus.gov, 8/26/17

Klosowski, T., "The Nutritional Differences Between Fresh and Frozen Food Explained," lifehacker.com, 11/17/13

Organic food is healthier than conventional food. Fact. p. 259

Chait, J., "Top Myths About Organic Food," thebalancesmb.com, 3/15/18

"Facts and Myths About Organic," greenblender.com, n.d.

"Impacts of Pesticides on Health," pan-uk.org, n.d.

Jackson-Michel, S., Dr., "The Effects of Herbicides & Pesticides on Humans," healthfully.com, 6/13/17

Nicolopoulou-Stamati, P., Maipas, S., Hens, L., "Chemical Pesticides and Human Health: The Urgent Need for a New Concept in Agriculture," ncbi.nlm.nih.gov, 7/18/16

Apple cider vinegar is a wonder food that can help with a number of ailments. Fact. p. 263

Colquhoun, J., "8 Proven Benefits of Apple Cider Vinegar," foodmatters.com, 8/25/15

Gunnars, K., BSc, "6 Health Benefits of Apple Cider Vinegar, Backed by Science," healthlinenutrition.com, 3/15/18

Sass, C., MPH, RD, "These Are The Real Health Benefits of Apple Cider Vinegar," health.com, 1/23/18

Bone broth is an overrated, so called health food, that is basically just soup. Myth. p. 265

Anderson, C.H., "8 Bone Broth Benefits That Will Convince You to Try the Trend," shape.com, 5/11/17

Axe, J., DNM, DC, CNS, *Bone Broth Breakthrough,* 2016

Geary, M., CNS, "The Healing Benefits of Delicious Bone Broth (for gut health and joint health)," nutritionwatchdog.com, July 2016

Shapiro, J., MD, "Bone Broth Benefits: Treat Leaky Gut, Reduce Cellulite and More!" doctorshealthpress.com, 3/17/16

Drinking red wine daily can help you live longer and lose weight. Fact. p. 268

"A Little Wine Each Day May Help Remove Waste From The Brain, Improve Cognitive Health, Research Finds," sciencenaturalnews.com, 2/15/18

Brazier, Y., Weatherspoon, D., PhD, RN, CRNA, "Is Red Wine Good For You?," medicalnewstoday.com, 9/7/17

Hamblin, J. "Wine and Exercise: A Promising Combination," theatlantic.com, 9/3/14

Stay away from beer unless you want a beer belly. Myth. p. 270

"Debunking the Myths Surrounding Dark Beers," craftbeer.com, 2/2/12

"Do Dark Beers Have More Alcohol Than Lighter Beers?" glacier-design.com, 8/6/17

Schatzker, M., "Top 5 Reasons to Drink Craft Beer," doctoroz.com, 4/16/18

Zelman, K.M., MPH, RD, LD, "The Truth About Beer and Your Belly," webmd.com, n.d.

Intermittent fasting is a fad and has no proven benefits. Myth. p. 274

Fung, Dr. J., MD, "How to Renew Your Body: Fasting and Autophagy," dietdoctor.com, October 2016

Gunnars, K., "10 Evidence-Based Health Benefits of Intermittent Fasting," healthline.com, 8/16/16

Sugarman, J., "Are There Any Proven Benefits of Fasting?" *Johns Hopkins Health Review,*
Volume 3/Issue 1, Spring/Summer 2016

"What the Science says About Intermittent Fasting," fitnessmercola.com, 6/28/13

Section Four

Sleep is more important than exercise and nutrition. Fact. p. 295

Carollo, L., "A Sleep Scientist on the Vicious Cycle of Insomnia and Sleeping Pills," thecut.com, 10/20/17

"Here's How Much Experts Think You Should Sleep Every Night," timeinc.net, 5/1/17

Leech, Joe, MS, "10 Reasons Why Sleep Is Important," healthline.com, 6/4/17

McIntosh, C., "Cultivate Better Sleep," *AARP Magazine,* Feb/Mar 2018

Sparacino, A., "11 Surprising Health Benefits of Sleep," health.com, 5/9/16

"Why Is Sleep Important?," nhlbi.nih.gov, 6/7/17

Our gut-brain connection is closely linked. Fact. p. 300

Komaroff, A., "The Gut-Brain Connection," health.harvard.edu, n.d.

Perlmutter, D., MD, *Brain Maker,* 2015

Robertson, R., PhD, "10 Ways to Improve Your Gut Bacteria, Based on Science," healthline.com, 11/18/16

"The Brain-Gut Connection," hopkinsmedicine.org, n.d.

Food cravings are mostly due to our emotional state. Fact. p. 303

Lawrence, J., "Do Food Cravings Reflect Your Feelings?" webmd.com, n.d.

Minich, D., Dr., "What the Nine Top Food Cravings Say About Your Emotion," deannaminich.com, 2/5/16

Winters, N., Dr., ND, Kelley, J.H., MNT, The *Metabolic Approach to Cancer,* 2017

Fluoride is safe for drinking water. Myth. p. 305

Connett, P., Dr., "50 Reasons to Oppose Fluoridation," fluoridealert.org, 4/12/04
Davis, N., PhD., "Is Fluoridated Drinking Water Safe?," hsps.harvard.edu, 6/15/16
Mercola, J., Dr., "10 Facts About Fluoride You Need to Know," articles.mercola.com, 4/30/13
Peckham, S., Awofeso, N., "Water Fluoridation: A Critical Review of the Physiological Effects of Ingested Fluoride as a Public Health Intervention," ncbi.nlm.nih.gov, 2/26/14

Calcium supplements are crucial for the health of your bones. Myth. p. 310

Dean, C., MD, ND, "Magnesium is Crucial for Bones," huffingtonpost.com, 8/15/12
Thompson, R., MD, *The Calcium Lie*, July 2013
Walker, R., Dr., "Myth: Calcium is Essential to Prevent Osteoporosis," medium.com, 2/25/18

Nutritional supplements are expensive and not beneficial if you are eating a balanced diet. Myth. p. 312

Axe, J., DNM, CNS, DC, "Should You Be Taking Magnesium Supplements?", "L-Glutamine Benefits Leaky Gut & Metabolism," draxe.com, 4/1/15
Leveque, K, "A Holistic Nutritionist on the Daily Supplements You Need Now," thechalkboardmag.com, 1/12/17
"Top Five Supplements Everyone Should Take," main.poliquingroup.com, 8/10/16

Meditation is an unproven therapy for mental and physical health. Myth. **p. 317**

Corliss, J., "Mindful Meditation May Ease Anxiety, Mental Stress," harvard.edu, 10/3/17

"Habits: How to Kickstart Your Healthy Day," healthiq.com, 2/20/18

"Meditation: Benefits for the Body," healthiq.com, 6/20/18

Sunshine at all levels is harmful and should be avoided unless sunblock is applied. Myth. **p. 322**

Dossantos, N., "15 Health Benefits of Sunshine," theactivetimes.com, 4/27/16

"Is Sunscreen Safe? What the Doc's Not Telling You," education.com, 5/2/14

Loux, R., "6 Scary Sunscreen Ingredients and 6 Safe SPF Products," womenshealth.com, 5/23/12

Mercola, J., ND, "Sunshine is Nature's Disease Fighter," articles.mercola.com, 7/3/08

Mercola, J., ND, "Why the Sun is Necessary for Optimal Health," articles.mercola.com, 10/15/16

Millions of Americans have parasites in them. Fact. **p. 327**

Firger, J., "CDC Warns of Common Parasites Plaguing Millions in U.S.," cbsnews.com, 5/8/14

Fox, M., "Rat Lungworm May Be More Common in U.S. than People Think," nbcnews.com, 8/2/18

Jockers, D., DC, MS, CSCS., "What Type of Parasites do You Have?" drjockers.com, n.d.

For the money, baking soda may be the healthiest, cheapest, and most versatile product on the market. Fact. p. 329

Axe, J., DNM, DC, CNS, "33 Surprising Baking Soda Uses and Remedies," draxe.com, n.d.

Lebow, H., "45 Cures of Baking Soda," thealternativedaily.com, 9/14/18

Marcin, J., MD, Cherney, K., "Can Store-Bought Baking Soda Really Treat Acid Reflux?" healthline.com, 9/16/16

Wilson, D., PhD, MSN, RN, IBCLC, AHN-BC, CHT, Leonard, J., "Baking Soda for Acid Reflux: Does it Work?" medicalnewstoday.com, 1/1/16

Epsom salt baths have astounding health benefits. Fact. p. 331

Butler, K., "6 Unexpected Health and Beauty Benefits of Epsom Salt," womenshealth.com, 3/1/16

DerSarkissian, C., "Why Take an Epsom Salt Bath?" webmd.com, 7/20/17

"Epsom Salt-The Magnesium-Rich Detoxifying Pain Reliever," draxe.com, n.d.

Some essential oils are more effective than antibiotics in fighting superbugs. Fact. p. 332

"Essential Oils Protection Against Superbugs," undergroundhealthreporter.com, n.d.

"Essential Oils to Fight Superbugs," Society for General Microbiology, sciencedaily.com, 4/4/10

Winters, N., ND, FABNO, L.Ac, Dipl.OM, Kelley, J.H., MNT, The *Metabolic Approach to Cancer,* 2017

Colors affect the human mind and body. Fact. p. 336

Editorial Staff, "Effect of Different Colors on Human Mind and Body," humannhealth.com, 10/5 13

"How Colors Manipulate Your Emotions," somer-somer.com, 3/30/15

Westland, S., "Here's How Colors Really Affect Our Brain and Body According to Science," sciencealert.com, 9/30/17

The color of a food indicates the healing properties within that food. Fact. p. 338

Jockers, D., DC, MS, CSCS., "The Unique Benefits of Eating Colorful Foods," drjockers.com, n.d.

Swartz, E., "Food and Color," healing-journeys-energy.com, 2006-2018

Templeton, H., "5 Ways to Decode Food's Health Benefits by Color," Food & Drink, mensjournal.com, n.d.

Would You Do Me A Favor?

Thank you for reading *Wellness Toolbox*. I hope you'll use what you've learned to feel, look, and perform better than you ever have before.

I have a small favor to ask...

Would you mind taking a minute to write a blurb on Amazon about this book? I check all my reviews and love to get honest feedback. That's the real joy for my work – knowing that I'm helping people.

To leave a review:

Pull up Amazon on your web browser; search for "Wellness Toolbox"; click on the book; scroll down and click on the "Write a Customer Review" button.

Thanks again, and I really look forward to reading your feedback.

Don

About the Author

Don Roberts is a fitness and nutrition specialist, group fitness instructor, public speaker, business consultant, and author. He is the founder, owner, and manager of Fit 24/7 gym (since 2002; a.k.a. Fitness Solutions 24/7), a vibrant and thriving business in Durango, Colorado, where he lives with his wife Teri and their two teenage boys.

In the health and fitness industry since 1991, Don has trained thousands of women and men of all ages, shapes, sizes, and abilities. He is well known for creating unique, fun, challenging, efficient, and effective training programs. Together with these fitness programs, Don's customized eating plans have helped hundreds of individuals attain healthy weight goals and improve their athletic performance. His portfolio is bursting with remarkable success stories and before/after photos of his clients.

Don's passion for exposing many myths and facts about both food and fitness is evident in his writing, public speaking, personal training, and nutritional consulting.

Don@Fit247Gym.com

www.Fit247Gym.com

Made in the USA
Middletown, DE
25 January 2023

21746588R00212